The
Cancer
Journals

Special Edition

Audre Lorde

aunt lute books

SAN FRANCISCO

Sections I and II of this book originally appeared in *Sinister Wisdom*.

aunt lute books
P. O. Box 410687
San Francisco, CA 94141

Cover Photo: Jean Weisinger
Cover Design: Electra Typography
Typesetter: Electra Typography

Senior Editor: Joan Pinkvoss
Managing Editor: Shay Brawn
Production: Tricia Lambie
          Norma Torres
          Christine Scudder
          Shivani Manghnani

ISBN 1-879960-51-6
Printed in the United States of America

Library of Congress Catologing-in-Publication Data

Lorde, Audre
    The cancer journals / Audre Lorde. — Special ed.
p. cm.
Includes bibliographical references (p.).
ISBN 1-879960-51-6

1. Lorde, Audre—Diaries. 2. Breast—Cancer—Patients—United
States—Biography. 3. Poets, American—20th century—Diaries.
I. Title.
RC280.B8L58   1997
362.1'9699449'0092—dc21
[B]   97-10954
                                     CIP

10 9 8 7 6 5 4 3 2

I wish to acknowledge with gratitude all the women who shared their strength with me throughout this time, and a special thanks to Maureen Brady, Frances Clayton, Michelle Cliff, Blanche Cook, Clare Coss, Judith McDaniel, and Adrienne Rich, whose loving support and criticisms helped bring this work to completion.

Introduction

1

Each woman responds to the crisis that breast cancer brings to her life out of a whole pattern, which is the design of who she is and how her life has been lived. The weave of her every day existence is the training ground for how she handles crisis. Some women obscure their painful feelings surrounding mastectomy with a blanket of business-as-usual, thus keeping those feelings forever under cover, but expressed elsewhere. For some women, in a valiant effort not to be seen as merely victims, this means an insistence that no such feelings exist and that nothing much has occurred. For some women it means the warrior's painstaking examination of yet another weapon, unwanted but useful.

I am a post-mastectomy woman who believes our feelings need voice in order to be recognized, respected, and of use.

I do not wish my anger and pain and fear about cancer to fossilize into yet another silence, nor to rob me of whatever strength can lie at the core of this experience, openly acknowledged and examined. For other women of all ages, colors, and sexual identities who recognize that imposed silence about any area of our lives is a tool for separation and powerlessness, and for myself, I have tried to voice some of my feelings and thoughts about the travesty of prosthesis, the pain of amputation, the function of cancer in a profit economy, my confrontation with mortality, the strength of women loving, and the power and rewards of self-conscious living.

Breast cancer and mastectomy are not unique experiences, but ones shared by thousands of american women. Each of these women has a particular voice to be raised in what must become a female outcry against all preventable cancers, as well as against the secret fears that allow those cancers to flourish. May these words serve as encouragement for other women to speak and to act out of our experiences with cancer and with other threats of death, for silence has never brought us anything of worth. Most of all, may these words underline the possibilities of self-healing and the richness of living for all women.

There is a commonality of isolation and painful reassessment which is shared by all women with breast cancer, whether this commonality is recognized or not. It is not my intention to judge the woman who has chosen the path of prosthesis, of silence and invisibility, the woman who wishes to be 'the same as before.' She has survived on another kind of courage, and she is not alone. Each of us struggles daily with the pressures of conformity and the loneliness of difference from which those choices seem to offer escape. I only know that those choices do not work for me, nor for other women who, not without fear, have survived cancer by scrutinizing its meaning within our lives, and by attempting to integrate this crisis into useful strengths for change.

2

These selected journal entries, which begin 6 months after my modified radical mastectomy for breast cancer and extend beyond the completion of the essays in this book, exemplify the process of integrating this crisis into my life.

1/26/79

I'm not feeling very hopeful these days, about selfhood or anything else. I handle the outward motions of each day while pain fills me like a puspocket and every touch threatens to breach the taut membrane that keeps it from flowing through and poisoning my whole existence. Sometimes despair sweeps across my consciousness like luna winds across a barren moonscape. Ironshod horses rage back and forth over every nerve. Oh Seboulisa ma, help me remember what I have paid so much to learn. I could die of difference, or live—myriad selves.

2/5/79

The terrible thing is that nothing goes past me these days, nothing. Each horror remains like a steel vise in my flesh, another magnet to the flame. Buster has joined the rolecall of useless wasteful deaths of young Black people; in the gallery today everywhere ugly images of women offering up distorted bodies for whatever fantasy passes in the name of male art. Gargoyles of pleasure. Beautiful laughing Buster, shot down in a hallway for ninety cents. Shall I unlearn that tongue in which my curse is written?

3/1/79

It is such an effort to find decent food in this place, not to just give up and eat the old poison. But I must tend my body with at least as much care as I tend the compost, particularly now when it seems so beside the point. Is this pain and despair that surround me a result of cancer, or has it just been released by cancer? I feel so unequal to what I always handled before, the abominations outside that echo the pain within. And yes I am completely self-referenced right now because it is the only translation I can trust, and I do believe not until every woman traces her weave back strand by bloody self-referenced strand, will we begin to alter the whole pattern.

4/16/79

The enormity of our task, to turn the world around. It feels like turning my life around, inside out. If I can look directly at my life and my death without flinching I know there is nothing they can ever do to me again. I must be content to see how really little I can do and still do it with an open heart. I can never accept this, like I can't accept that turning my life around is so hard, eating differently, sleeping differently, moving differently, being differently. Like Martha said, I want the old me, bad as before.

4/22/79

I must let this pain flow through me and pass on. If I resist or try to stop it, it will detonate inside me, shatter me, splatter my pieces against every wall and person that I touch.

5/1/79

Spring comes, and still I feel despair like a pale cloud waiting to consume me, engulf me like another cancer, swallow me into immobility, metabolize me into cells of itself; my body, a barometer. I need to remind myself of the joy, the lightness, the laughter so vital to my living and my health. Otherwise, the other will always be waiting to eat me up into despair again. And that means destruction. I don't know how, but it does.

9/79

There is no room around me in which to be still, to examine and explore what pain is mine alone—no device to separate my struggle within from my fury at the outside world's viciousness, the stupid brutal lack of consciousness or concern that passes for the way things are. The arrogant blindness of comfortable white women. What is this work all for? What does it matter whether I ever speak again or not? I try. The blood of black women sloshes from coast to coast and Daly says race is of no concern to women. So that means we are either immortal or born to die and no note taken, un-women.

10/3/79

I don't feel like being strong, but do I have a choice? It hurts when even my sisters look at me in the street with cold and silent eyes. I am defined as other in every group I'm a part of. The outsider, both strength and weakness. Yet without community there is certainly no liberation, no future, only the most vulnerable and temporary armistice between me and my oppression.

11/19/79

I want to write rage but all that comes is sadness. We have been sad long enough to make this earth either weep or grow fertile. I am an anachronism, a sport, like the bee that was never meant to fly. Science said so. I am not supposed to exist. I carry death around in my body like a condemnation. But I do live. The bee flies. There must be some way to integrate death into living, neither ignoring it nor giving in to it.

1/1/80

Faith is the last day of Kwanza, and the name of the war against despair, the battle I fight daily. I become better at it. I want to write about that battle, the skirmishes, the losses, the small yet so important victories that make the sweetness of my life.

1/20/80

The novel is finished at last. It has been a lifeline. I do not have to win in order to know my dreams are valid, I only have to believe in a process of which I am a part. My work kept me alive this past year, my work and the love of women. They are inseparable from each other. In the recognition of the existence of love lies the answer to despair. Work is that recognition given voice and name.

2/18/80

I am 46 years living today and very pleased to be alive, very glad and very happy. Fear and pain and despair do not disappear. They only become slowly less and less important. Although sometimes I still long for a simple orderly life with a hunger sharp as that sudden vegetarian hunger for meat.

4/6/80

Somedays, if bitterness were a whetstone, I could be sharp as grief.

5/30/80

Last spring was another piece of the fall and winter before, a progression from all the pain and sadness of that time, ruminated over. But somehow this summer which is almost upon me feels like a part of my future. Like a brand new time, and I'm pleased to know it, wherever it leads. I feel like another woman, de-chrysalised and become a broader, stretched-out me, strong and excited, a muscle flexed and honed for action.

6/20/80

I do not forget cancer for very long, ever. That keeps me armed and on my toes, but also with a slight background noise of fear. Carl Simonton's book, Getting Well Again, *has been really helpful to me, even though his smugness infuriates me sometimes. The visualizations and deep relaxing techniques that I learned from it help make me a less anxious person, which seems strange, because in other ways, I live with the constant fear of recurrence of another cancer. But fear and anxiety are not the same at all. One is an appropriate response to a real situation which I can accept and learn to work through just as I work through semi-blindness. But the other, anxiety, is an immobilizing yield to things that go bump in the night, a surrender to namelessness, formlessness, voicelessness, and silence.*

7/10/80

I dreamt I had begun training to change my life, with a teacher who is very shadowy. I was not attending classes, but I was going to learn how to change my whole life, live differently, do everything in a new and different way. I didn't really understand, but I trusted this shadowy teacher. Another young woman who was there told me she was taking a course in "language crazure," the opposite of discrazure (the cracking and wearing away of rock). I thought it would be very exciting to study the formation and crack and composure of words, so I told my teacher I wanted to take that course. My teacher said okay, but it wasn't going to help me any because I had to learn something else, and I wouldn't get anything new from that class. I replied maybe not, but even though I knew all about rocks, for instance, I still liked studying their composition, and giving a name to the different ingredients of which they were made. It's very exciting to think of me being all the people in this dream.

3

I have learned much in the 18 months since my mastectomy. My visions of a future I can create have been honed by the lessons of my limitations. Now I wish to give form with honesty and precision to the pain faith labor and loving which this period of my life has translated into strength for me.

Sometimes fear stalks me like another malignancy, sapping energy and power and attention from my work. A cold becomes sinister; a cough, lung cancer; a bruise, leukemia. Those fears are most powerful when they are not given voice, and close upon their heels comes the fury that I cannot shake them. I am learning to live beyond fear by living through it, and in the process learning to turn fury at my own limitations into some more creative energy. I realize that if I wait until I am no longer afraid to act, write, speak, be, I'll be sending messages on a Ouija board, cryptic complaints from the other side. When l dare to be powerful, to use my strength in the service of my vision, then it becomes less important whether or not I am unafraid.

As women we were raised to fear. If I cannot banish fear completely, I can learn to count with it less. For then fear becomes not a tyrant against which I waste my energy fighting, but a companion, not particularly desirable, yet one whose knowledge can be useful.

I write so much here about fear because in shaping this introduction to *The Cancer Journals*, I found fear laid across my hands like a steel bar. When I tried to reexamine the 18 months since my mastectomy, some of what I touched was molten despair and waves of mourning—for my lost breast, for time, for the luxury of false power. Not only were these emotions difficult and painful to relive, but they were entwined with the terror that if I opened myself once again to scrutiny, to feeling the pain of loss, of despair, of victories too minor in my eyes to rejoice over, then I might also open myself again to disease. I had to remind myself that I had lived through it all, already. I had known the pain, and survived it. It only remained for me to give it voice, to share it for use, that the pain not be wasted.

Living a self-conscious life, under the pressure of time, I work with the consciousness of death at my shoulder, not constantly, but often enough to leave a mark upon all of my life's decisions and actions. And it does not matter whether this death comes next week or thirty years from now; this consciousness gives my life another breadth. It helps shape the words I speak, the ways I love, my politic of action, the strength of my vision and purpose, the depth of my appreciation of living.

I would lie if I did not also speak of loss. Any amputation is a physical and psychic reality that must be integrated into a new sense of self. The absence of my breast is a recurrent sadness, but certainly not one that dominates my life. I miss it, sometimes piercingly. When other one-breasted women hide behind the mask of prosthesis or the dangerous fantasy of reconstruction, I find little support in the broader female environment for my rejection of what feels like a cosmetic sham. But I believe that socially sanctioned prosthesis is merely another way of keeping women with breast cancer silent and separate from each other. For instance, what would happen if an army of one-breasted women descended upon Congress and demanded that the use of carcinogenic, fat-stored hormones in beef-feed be outlawed?

The lessons of the past 18 months have been many: How do I provide myself with the best physical and psychic nourishment to repair past, and minimize future damage to my body? How do I give voice to my quests so that other women can take what they need from my experiences? How do my experiences with cancer fit into the larger tapestry of my work as a Black woman, into the history of all women? And most of all, how do I fight the despair born of fear and anger and powerlessness which is my greatest internal enemy?

I have found that battling despair does not mean closing my eyes to the enormity of the tasks of effecting change, nor ignoring the strength and the barbarity of the forces aligned against us. It means teaching, surviving and fighting with the most important resource I have, myself, and taking joy in that battle. It means, for me, recognizing the enemy outside, and the enemy within, and knowing that my work is part of a continuum of women's work, of reclaiming this earth and our power, and knowing that this work did not begin with my birth nor will it end with my death. And it means knowing that within this continuum, my life and my love and my work has particular power and meaning relative to others.

It means trout fishing on the Missisquoi River at dawn and tasting the green silence, and knowing that this beauty too is mine forever.

29 August 1980

I

The Transformation of Silence into Language and Action*

I would like to preface my remarks on the transformation of silence into language and action with a poem. The title of it is "A Song for Many Movements" and this reading is dedicated to Winnie Mandela. Winnie Mandela is a South African freedom fighter who is in exile now somewhere in South Africa. She had been in prison and had been released and was picked up again after she spoke out against the recent jailing of black school children who were singing freedom songs, and who were charged with public violence…"A Song for Many Movements":

> Nobody wants to die on the way
> caught between ghosts of whiteness
> and the real water
> none of us wanted to leave
> our bones
> on the way to salvation

*Originally given as a speech, December 28, 1977, at the Lesbian and Literature Panel of the Modern Language Association.

three planets to the left
a century of light years ago
our spices are separate and particular
but our skins sing in complimentary keys
at a quarter to eight mean time
we were telling the same stories
over and over and over.

Broken down gods survive
in the crevasses and mudpots
of every beleaguered city
where it is obvious
there are too many bodies
to cart to the ovens
or gallows
and our uses have become
more important than our silence
after the fall
too many empty cases
of blood to bury or burn
there will be no body left
to listen
and our labor
has become more important
than our silence.

Our labor has become
more important
than our silence.

(from Audre Lorde's *The Black Unicorn*, W.W. Norton & Co., 1978)

I have come to believe over and over again that what is
most important to me must be spoken, made verbal and
shared, even at the risk of having it bruised or misunderstood.
That the speaking profits me, beyond any other effect. I am

standing here as a black lesbian poet, and the meaning of all that waits upon the fact that I am still alive, and might not have been. Less than two months ago, I was told by two doctors, one female and one male, that I would have to have breast surgery, and that there was a 60 to 80 percent chance that the tumor was malignant. Between that telling and the actual surgery, there was a three week period of the agony of an involuntary reorganization of my entire life. The surgery was completed, and the growth was benign.

But within those three weeks, I was forced to look upon myself and my living with a harsh and urgent clarity that has left me still shaken but much stronger. This is a situation faced by many women, by some of you here today. Some of what I experienced during that time has helped elucidate for me much of what I feel concerning the transformation of silence into language and action.

In becoming forcibly and essentially aware of my mortality, and of what I wished and wanted for my life, however short it might be, priorities and omissions became strongly etched in a merciless light, and what I most regretted were my silences. Of what had I *ever* been afraid? To question or to speak as I believed could have meant pain, or death. But we all hurt in so many different ways, all the time, and pain will either change, or end. Death, on the other hand, is the final silence. And that might be coming quickly, now, without regard for whether I had ever spoken what needed to be said, or had only betrayed myself into small silences, while I planned someday to speak, or waited for someone else's words. And I began to recognize a source of power within myself that comes from the knowledge that while it is most desirable not to be afraid, learning to put fear into a perspective gave me great strength.

I was going to die, if not sooner then later, whether or not I had ever spoken myself. My silences had not protected me. Your silence will not protect you. But for every real word spoken, for every attempt I had ever made to speak those truths for which I am still seeking, I had made contact with other women while we examined the words to fit a world in which we all believed, bridging our differences. And it was the concern and caring of all those women which gave me strength and enabled me to scrutinize the essentials of my living.

The women who sustained me through that period were black and white, old and young, lesbian, bisexual, and heterosexual, and we all shared a war against the tyrannies of silence. They all gave me a strength and concern without which I could not have survived intact. Within those weeks of acute fear came the knowledge—within the war we are all waging with the forces of death, subtle and otherwise, conscious or not—I am not only a casualty, I am also a warrior.

What are the words you do not yet have? What do you need to say? What are the tyrannies you swallow day by day and attempt to make your own, until you will sicken and die of them, still in silence? Perhaps for some of you here today, I am the face of one of your fears. Because I am woman, because I am black, because I am lesbian, because I am myself, a black woman warrior poet doing my work, come to ask you, are you doing yours?

And, of course, I am afraid—you can hear it in my voice—because the transformation of silence into language and action is an act of self-revelation and that always seems fraught with danger. But my daughter, when I told her of our topic and my difficulty with it, said, "Tell them about how you're never really a whole person if you remain silent, because there's always that one little piece inside of you that wants to be spoken out, and if you keep ignoring it, it gets madder and madder and hotter and hotter, and if you don't speak it out one day it will just up and punch you in the mouth."

In the cause of silence, each one of us draws the face of her own fear—fear of contempt, of censure, or some judgment, or recognition, of challenge, of annihilation. But most of all, I think, we fear the very visibility without which we also cannot truly live. Within this country where racial difference creates a constant, if unspoken, distortion of vision, black women have on one hand always been highly visible, and so, on the other hand, have been rendered invisible through the depersonalization of racism. Even within the women's movement, we have had to fight and still do, for that very visibility which also renders us most vulnerable, our blackness. For to survive in the mouth of this dragon we call america, we have had to learn this first and most vital lesson—that we were never meant to survive. Not as human beings. And neither were most of you here today, black or not. And that visibility which makes us most vulnerable is that which also is the source of our greatest strength. Because the machine will try to grind you into dust anyway, whether or not we speak. We can sit in our corners mute forever while our sisters and our selves are wasted, while our children are distorted and destroyed, while our earth is poisoned, we can sit in our safe corners mute as bottles, and we still will be no less afraid.

In my house this year we are celebrating the feast of Kwanza, the African-American festival of harvest which begins the day after Christmas and lasts for seven days. There are seven principles of Kwanza, one for each day. The first principle is Umoja, which means unity, the decision to strive for and maintain unity in self and community. The principle for yesterday, the second day, was Kujichagulia—self-determination—the decision to define ourselves, name ourselves, and speak for ourselves, instead of being defined and spoken for by others. Today is the third day of Kwanza, and the principle for today is Ujima—collective work and responsibility—the decision to build and maintain ourselves and our communities together and to recognize and solve our problems together.

Each of us is here now because in one way or another we share a commitment to language and to the power of language, and to the reclaiming of that language which has been made to work against us. In the transformation of silence into language and action, it is vitally necessary for each one of us to establish or examine her function in that transformation, and to recognize her role as vital within that transformation.

For those of us who write, it is necessary to scrutinize not only the truth of what we speak, but the truth of that language by which we speak it. For others, it is to share and spread also those words that are meaningful to us. But primarily for us all, it is necessary to teach by living and speaking those truths which we believe and know beyond understanding. Because in this way alone we can survive, by taking part in a process of life that is creative and continuing, that is growth.

And it is never without fear; of visibility, of the harsh light of scrutiny and perhaps judgment, of pain, of death. But we have lived through all of those already, in silence, except death. And I remind myself all the time now, that if I were to have been born mute, or had maintained an oath of silence my whole life long for safety, I would still have suffered, and I would still die. It is very good for establishing perspective.

And where the words of women are crying to be heard, we must each of us recognize our responsibility to seek those words out, to read them and share them and examine them in their pertinence to our lives. That we not hide behind the mockeries of separations that have been imposed upon us and which so often we accept as our own: for instance, "I can't possibly teach black women's writing—their experience is so different from mine," yet how many years have you spent teaching Plato and Shakespeare and Proust? Or another: "She's a white woman and what could she possibly have to say to me?" Or, "She's a lesbian, what would my husband say, or my chairman?" Or again, "This woman writes of her sons and I have no children." And all the other endless ways in which we rob ourselves of ourselves and each other.

We can learn to work and speak when we are afraid in the

same way we have learned to work and speak when we are tired. For we have been socialized to respect fear more than our own needs for language and definition, and while we wait in silence for that final luxury of fearlessness, the weight of that silence will choke us.

The fact that we are here and that I speak now these words is an attempt to break that silence and bridge some of those differences between us, for it is not difference which immobilizes us, but silence. And there are so many silences to be broken.

II

Breast Cancer:
A Black Lesbian Feminist Experience

March 25, 1978

The idea of knowing, rather than believing, trusting, or even under-standing has always been considered heretical. But I would willingly pay whatever price in pain was needed, to savor the weight of comple-tion; to be utterly filled, not with conviction nor with faith, but with experience—knowledge, direct and different from all other certainties.

October 10, 1978

I want to write about the pain. The pain of waking up in the recovery room which is worsened by that immediate sense of loss. Of going in and out of pain and shots. Of the correct position for my arm to drain. The euphoria of the 2nd day, and how it's been downhill from there.

I want to write of the pain I am feeling right now, of the lukewarm tears that will not stop coming into my eyes—for what? For my lost breast? For the lost me? And which me was that again anyway? For the death I don't know how to postpone? Or how to meet elegantly?

I'm so tired of all this. I want to be the person I used to be, the real me. I feel sometimes that it's all a dream and surely I'm about to wake up now.

November 2, 1978

How do you spend your time, she said. Reading, mostly, I said. I couldn't tell her that mostly I sat staring at blank walls, or getting stoned into my heart, and then, one day when I found I could finally masturbate again, making love to myself for hours at a time. The flame was dim and flickering, but it was a welcome relief to the long coldness.

December 29, 1978

What is there possibly left for us to be afraid of, after we have dealt face to face with death and not embraced it? Once I accept the existence of dying, as a life process, who can ever have power over me again?

This is work I must do alone. For months now I have been wanting to write a piece of meaning words on cancer as it affects my life and my consciousness as a woman, a black lesbian feminist mother lover poet all I am. But even more, or the same, I want to illuminate the implications of breast cancer for me, and the threats to self-revelation that are so quickly aligned against any woman who seeks to explore those questions, those answers. Even in the face of our own deaths and dignity, we are not to be allowed to define our needs nor our feelings nor our lives.

I could not even write about the outside threats to my vision and action because the inside pieces were too frightening.

This reluctance is a reluctance to deal with myself, with my own experiences and the feelings buried in them, and the conclusions to be drawn from them. It is also, of course, a reluctance to living or re-living, giving life or new life to that pain. The pain of separation from my breast was at least as sharp as the pain of separating from my mother. But I made it once before, so I know I can make it again.

Trying to even set this all down step by step is a process of focussing in from the periphery towards the center.

A year ago I was told I had an 80% chance of having breast cancer. That time, the biopsy was negative. But in that interim of three weeks between being told that I might have cancer and finding out it was not so, I met for the first time the essential questions of my own mortality. I was going to die, and it might be a lot sooner than I had ever conceived of. That knowledge did not disappear with the diagnosis of a benign tumor. If not now, I told my lover, then someday. None of us have 300 years. The terror that I conquered in those three weeks left me with a determination and freedom to speak as I needed, and to enjoy and live my life as I needed to for my own meaning.

During the next summer, the summer of 1978, I wrote in my journal:

> *Whatever the message is, may I survive the delivery of it. Is letting go a process or a price? What am I paying for, not seeing sooner? Learning at the edge? Letting go of something precious but no longer needed?*

So this fall I met cancer, as it were, from a considered position, but it still knocked me for a hell of a loop, having to deal with the pain and the fear and the death I thought I had come to terms with once before. I did not recognize then how many faces those terms had, nor how many forces were aligned within our daily structures against them, nor how often I would have to redefine the terms because other experiences kept presenting themselves. The acceptance of death as a fact, rather than the desire to die, can empower my energies with a forcefulness and vigor not always possible when one eye is out unconsciously for eternity.

Last month, three months after surgery, I wrote in my journal:

I seem to move so much more slowly now these days. It is as if I cannot do the simplest thing, as if nothing at all is done without a decision, and every decision is so crucial. Yet I feel strong and able in general, and only sometimes do I touch that battered place where I am totally inadequate to any thing I most wish to accomplish. To put it another way, I feel always tender in the wrong places.

In September 1978, I went into the hospital for a breast biopsy for the second time. It all happened much faster this time than the year before. There was none of the deep dread of the previous biopsy, but at the same time there was none of the excitement of a brand new experience. I said to my surgeon the night before—"I'm a lot more scared this time, but I'm handling it better." On the surface, at least, we all expected it to be a repeat. My earlier response upon feeling this lump had been "I've been through this once before. What do we do for encore?"

Well, what we did for encore was the real thing.

I woke up in the recovery room after the biopsy colder than I can remember ever having been in my life. I was hurting and horrified. I knew it was malignant. How, I didn't know, but I suspect I had absorbed that fact from the operating room while I still was out. Being "out" really means only that you can't answer back or protect yourself from what you are absorbing through your ears and other senses. But when I raised my hand in the recovery room and touched both bandaged breasts, I knew there was a malignancy in one, and the other had been biopsied also. It was only for affirmation. I would have given anything to have been warmer right then. The gong in my brain of "malignant," "malignant," and the icy sensations of that frigid room, cut through the remnants of anesthesia like a fire hose trained on my brain. All I could focus upon was getting out of that room and getting warm. I yelled and screamed and complained about the cold and begged for extra blankets, but none came. The nurses were very put out by my ruckus and sent me back to the floor early.

My doctor had said he would biopsy both breasts if one was malignant. I couldn't believe this hospital couldn't shut off the air-conditioning or give me more blankets. The Amazon girls were only 15, I thought, how did they handle it?

Frances was there by the door of my room like a great sunflower. I surfaced from anesthesia again as she took my hand in her deliciously warm ones, her dear face bent over mine. "It is malignant, isn't it, Frances, it is malignant," I said. She squeezed my hand and I saw tears in her eyes. "Yes, my love, it is," she said, and the anesthesia washed out of me again before the sharp edge of fact. "Baby, I'm so cold, so cold," I said. The night before I had said to her, crying, before she left, "The real victory will be my waking up out of the anesthetic."

The decisions seemed much easier. The whole rest of that day seemed a trip back and forth through the small pain in both breasts and my acute awareness of the fact of death in the right one. This was mixed with the melting and chewing over of the realities, between Frances and me. Our comforting each other— "We'll make it through this together"—and the cold, the terrible cold of that first hour. And between us both, our joint tears, our rich loving. I swam in and out of sleep, mostly out.

Our friends came and were there, loving and helpful and there, brought coats to pile upon my bed and then a comforter and blankets because the hospital had no spare blankets, they said, and I was so desperately chilled from the cold recovery room.

I remember their faces as we shared the knowledge and the promise of shared strength in the trial days to come. In some way it was as if each of the people I love most dearly came one by one to my bedside where we made a silent pledge of strength and sisterhood no less sacred than if it had been pledged in blood rather than love.

Off and on I kept thinking. I have cancer. I'm a black lesbian feminist poet, how am I going to do this now? Where are the models for what I'm supposed to be in this situation? But there were none. This is it, Audre. You're on your own.

In the next two days, I came to realize as I agonized over my choices and what to do, that I had made my decision to have surgery if it were needed even before the biopsy had been done. Yet I had wanted a two-stage operation anyway, separating the biopsy from the mastectomy. I wanted time to re-examine my decision, to search really for some other alternative that would give me good reasons to change my mind. But there were none to satisfy me.

I wanted to make the decision again, and I did, knowing the other possibilities, and reading avidly and exhaustively through the books I ordered through Frances and Helen and my friends. These books now piled up everywhere in that wretched little room, making it at least a little bit like home.

Even before the biopsy, from the time I was admitted into the hospital Monday afternoon, the network of woman support had been begun by our friends. Blanche and Clare arrived from Southampton just in time before visiting hours were over bearing a gorgeous French rum and mocha cake with a marzipan banner that said 'we love you, audre,' outrageously rich and sinfully delicious. When the findings were malignant on Tuesday, this network swung into high gear. To this day, I don't know what Frances and I and the children would have done without it.

From the time I woke up to the slow growing warmth of Adrienne's and Bernice's and Deanna's and Michelle's and Frances' coats on the bed, I felt Beth Israel Hospital wrapped in a web of woman love and strong wishes of faith and hope for the whole time I was there, and it made self-healing more possible, knowing I was not alone. Throughout the hospitalization and for some time after, it seemed that no problem was too small or too large to be shared and handled.

My daughter Beth cried in the waiting room after I told her I was going to have a mastectomy. She said she was sentimentally attached to my breasts. Adrienne comforted her, somehow making Beth understand that hard as this was, it was different for me from if I had been her age, and that our experiences were different.

Adrienne offered to rise early to park the car for Frances so she could be with me before the operation. Blanche and Clare took the children shopping for school clothes, and helped give them a chance to cut up and laugh in the midst of all this grimness. My sister Helen made chicken soup with homemade dumplings. Bernice gathered material and names and addresses and testimonials for alternative treatments for breast cancer. And through those three days between the biopsy and the mastectomy, good wishes came pouring in by mail and telephone and the door and the psychic ether.

To this day, sometimes I feel like a corporate effort, the love and care and concern of so many women having been invested in me with such open-heartedness. My fears were the fears of us all.

And always, there was Frances, glowing with a steady warm light close by to the island within which I had to struggle alone.

I considered the alternatives of the straight medical profession, surgery, radiation, and chemotherapy. I considered the holistic health approaches of diet, vitamin therapy, experimental immunotherapeutics, west german pancreatic enzymes, and others. The decision whether or not to have a mastectomy ultimately was going to have to be my own. I had always been firm on that point and had chosen a surgeon with that in mind. With the various kinds of information I had gathered together before I went into the hospital, and the additional information acquired in the hectic three days after biopsy, now more than ever before I had to examine carefully the pros and cons of every possibility, while being constantly and acutely aware that so much was still not known.

And all the time as a background of pain and terror and disbelief, a thin high voice was screaming that none of this was true, it was all a bad dream that would go away if I became totally inert. Another part of me flew like a big bird to the ceiling of whatever place I was in, observing my actions and providing a running commentary, complete with suggestions of factors forgotten, new possibilities of movement, and ribald remarks. I felt as if I was always listening to a concert of voices from inside myself, all with something slightly different to say, all of which were quite insistent and none of which would let me rest.

They very effectively blotted out the other thin high voice that counseled sleep, but I still knew it was there, and sometimes in the middle of the night when I couldn't sleep, I wondered if perhaps it was not the voice of wisdom rather than despair.

I now realize that I was in a merciful state akin to shock in those days. In a sense it was my voices—those myriad pieces of myself and my background and experience and definitions of myself I had fought so long and hard to nourish and maintain—which were guiding me on automatic, so to speak. But it did not feel so at the time. I felt sometimes utterly calm cool and collected, as if this whole affair was an intellectual problem to be considered and solved: should I have a mastectomy or not? What was the wisest approach to take having a diagnosis of breast cancer and a history of cystic mastitis? Other times, I felt almost overwhelmed by pain and fury, and the inadequacies of my tools to make any meaningful decision, and yet I had to.

I was helped by the fact that one strong voice kept insisting that I had in truth made this decision already, all I had to do was remember the pieces and put them together. That used to annoy me sometimes, the feeling that I had less to decide than to remember.

I knew the horror that I had lived with for a year since my last biopsy had now become a reality, and in a sense that reality, however difficult, was easier to deal with than fear. But it was still very hard for me not only to face the idea of my own fragile mortality, but to anticipate more physical pain and the loss of such a cherished part of me as my breast. And all these things were operating at the same time I was having to make a decision as to what I should do. Luckily, I had been in training for a long time.

I listened to my voices, considered the alternatives, chewed over the material that concerned women brought to me. It seems like an eternity went by between my returning from the biopsy and my making a decision, but actually it was only a day and a half.

On Wednesday afternoon I told Frances that I had decided to have surgery, and tears came to her eyes. Later she told me that she had been terrified that I might refuse surgery, opting instead for an alternative treatment, and she felt that she was prepared to go along with whatever I would decide, but she also felt surgery was the wisest choice.

A large factor in this decision was the undeniable fact that any surgical intervention in a cystic area can possibly activate cancer cells that might otherwise remain dormant. I had dealt with that knowledge a year ago when deciding whether or not to have a biopsy, and with the probabilities of a malignancy being as high as they were then, I felt then I had no choice but to decide as I did. Now, I had to consider again whether surgery might start another disease process. I deluged my surgeon with endless questions which he answered in good faith, those that he could. I weighed my options. There were malignant cells in my right breast encased in a fatty cyst, and if I did not do something about that I would die of cancer in fairly short order. Whatever I did might or might not reverse that process, and I would not know with any certainty for a very long time.

When it came right down to deciding, as I told Frances later, I felt inside myself for what I really felt and wanted, and that was to live and to love and to do my work, as hard as I could and for as long as I could. So I simply chose the course that I felt most likely to achieve my desire, knowing that I would have paid more than even my beloved breast out of my body to preserve that self that was not merely physically defined, and count it well spent.

Having made that decision, I felt comfortable with it and able to move on. I could not choose the option of radiation and chemotherapy because I felt strongly that everything I had read about them suggested that they were in and of themselves carcinogenic. The experimental therapies without surgery were interesting possibilities, but still unproven. Surgery, a modified radical mastectomy, while traumatic and painful would arrest any process by removal. It was not in and of itself harmful at this point, since whatever process might have been started by surgery had already been begun by the biopsy. I knew that there might come a time when it was clear that surgery had been unnecessary because of the efficacy of alternate therapies. I might be losing my breast in vain. But nothing else was as sure, and it was a price I was willing to pay for life, and I felt I had chosen the wisest course for me. I think now what was most important was not what I chose to do so much as that I was conscious of being able to choose, and having chosen, was empowered from having made a decision, done a strike for myself, moved.

Throughout the three days between the mastectomy and the biopsy I felt positively possessed by a rage to live that became an absolute determination to do whatever was necessary to accomplish that living, and I remember wondering if I was strong enough to sustain that determination after I left the hospital. If I left the hospital. For all the deciding and great moral decisions going on, I was shit-scared about another bout with anesthesia. Familiarity with the procedures had not lessened my terror.

I was also afraid that I was not really in control, that it might already be too late to halt the spread of cancer, that there was simply too much to do that I might not get done, that the pain would be just too great. Too great for what, I did not know. I was afraid. That I would not survive another anesthesia, that the payment of my breast would not be enough; for what? Again, I did not know. I think perhaps I was afraid to continue being myself.

The year before, as I waited almost four weeks for my first biopsy, I had grown angry at my right breast because I felt as if it had in some unexpected way betrayed me, as if it had become already separate from me and had turned against me by creating this tumor which might be malignant. My beloved breast had suddenly departed from the rules we had agreed upon to function by all these years.

But on the day before my mastectomy I wrote in my journal:

September 21, 1978

> *The anger that I felt for my right breast last year has faded, and I'm glad because I have had this extra year. My breasts have always been so very precious to me since I accepted having them it would have been a shame not to have enjoyed the last year of one of them. And I think I am prepared to lose it now in a way I was not quite ready to last November, because now I really see it as a choice between my breast and my life, and in that view there cannot be any question.*
>
> *Somehow I always knew this would be the final outcome, for it never did seem like a finished business for me. This year between was like a hiatus, an interregnum in*

a battle within which I could so easily be a casualty, since I certainly was a warrior. And in that brief time the sun shone and the birds sang and I wrote important words and have loved richly and been loved in return. And if a lifetime of furies is the cause of this death in my right breast, there is still nothing I've never been able to accept before that I would accept now in order to keep my breast. It was a 12 month reprieve in which I could come to accept the emotional fact/truths I came to see first in those horrendous weeks last year before the biopsy. If I do what I need to do because I want to do it, it will matter less when death comes, because it will have been an ally that spurred me on.

I was relieved when the first tumor was benign, but I said to Frances at the time that the true horror would be if they said it was benign and it wasn't. I think my body knew there was a malignancy there somewhere, and that it would have to be dealt with eventually. Well, I'm dealing with it as best I can. I wish I didn't have to, and I don't even know if I'm doing it right, but I sure am glad that I had this extra year to learn to love me in a different way.

I'm going to have the mastectomy, knowing there are alternatives, some of which sound very possible in the sense of right thinking, but none of which satisfy me enough.... Since it is my life that I am gambling with, and my life is worth even more than the sensual delights of my breast, I certainly can't take that chance.

7:30 p.m. And yet if I cried for a hundred years I couldn't possibly express the sorrow I feel right now, the sadness and the loss. How did the Amazons* of Dahomey feel? They were only little girls. But they did this willingly, for something they believed in. I suppose I am too but I can't feel that now.

---

*It is said that the Amazon warriors of Dahomey have their right breasts cut off to make themselves more effective archers.

Eudora Garrett was not the first woman with whom I had shared body warmth and wildness, but she was the first woman who totally engaged me in our loving. I remember the hesitation and tenderness I felt as I touched the deeply scarred hollow under her right shoulder and across her chest, the night she finally shared the last pain of her mastectomy with me in the clear heavy heat of our Mexican spring. I was 19 and she was 47. Now I am 44 and she is dead.

Eudora came to me in my sleep that night before surgery in that tiny cold hospital room so different from her bright hot dishevelled bedroom in Cuernavaca, with her lanky snap-dragon self and her gap-toothed lopsided smile, and we held hands for a while.

The next morning before Frances came I wrote in my journal:

September 22, 1978
Today is the day in the grim rainy morning and all I can do now is weep, Eudora, what did I give you in those Mexican days so long ago ? Did you know how I loved you? You never talked of your dying, only of your work.

Then through the dope of tranquilizers and grass I remember Frances' hand on mine, and the last sight of her dear face like a great sunflower in the sky. There is the horror of those flashing lights passing over my face, and the clanging of disemboweled noises that have no context nor relationship to me except they assault me. There is the dispatch with which I have ceased being a person who is myself and become a thing upon a Guerney cart to be delivered up to Moloch, a dark living sacrifice in the white place.

I remember screaming and cursing with pain in the recovery room, and I remember a disgusted nurse giving me a shot. I remember a voice telling me to be quiet because there were sick people here, and my saying, well, I have a right, because

I'm sick too. Until 5:00 a.m. the next morning, waking was brief seas of localized and intense pain between shots and sleep. At 5:00 a nurse rubbed my back again, helped me get up and go to the bathroom because I couldn't use the bedpan, and then helped me into a chair. She made me a cup of tea and some fruit juice because I was parched. The pain had subsided a good deal.

I could not move my right arm nor my shoulder, both of which were numb, and wrapped around my chest was a wide Ace bandage under which on my left side the mound of my left breast arose, and from which on the right side protruded the ends of white surgical bandages. From under the Ace bandage on my right side, two plastic tubes emerged, running down into a small disc-shaped plastic bottle called a hemovac which drained the surgical area. I was alive, and it was a very beautiful morning. I drank my tea slowly, and then went back to bed.

I woke up again at about 7:30 to smell Frances outside my door. I couldn't see her because the sides of my bed were still up, but I sat up as best I could one-armed, and peeped around the corner and there she was, the person I needed and wanted most to see, and our smiles met each other's and bounced around the room and out into the corridor where they warmed up the whole third floor.

The next day the sun shone brilliantly, and for ten days steadily thereafter. The autumn equinox came—the middle—the sun now equidistant, then going away. It was one of those rare and totally gorgeous blue New York City autumns.

That next day after the operation was an incredible high. I now think of it as the euphoria of the second day. The pain was minimal. I was alive. The sun was shining. I remember feeling a little simple but rather relieved it was all over, or so I thought. I stuck a flower in my hair and thought "This is not as bad as I was afraid of."

During the first two days after surgery, I shared thanksgiving with beautiful and beloved women and slept. I remember the children coming to visit me and Beth joking, but how both of their faces were light with relief to see me so well. I felt as if there was grey smoke in my head and something I wasn't dealing with, but I wasn't sure what. Once I put a flower in my hair and walked through the halls looking for Frances who had gone into the waiting room with Michelle and Adrienne to let me rest.

From time to time I would put my hand upon the flattish mound of bandages on the right side of my chest and say to myself—my right breast is gone, and I would shed a few tears if I was alone. But I had no real emotional contact yet with the reality of the loss; it was as if I had been emotionally anesthetized also, or as if the only feelings I could reach were physical ones, and the scar was not only hidden under bandages but as yet was feeling little pain. When I looked at myself in the mirror even, the difference was not at all striking, because of the bulkiness of the bandages.

And my friends, who flooded me with love and concern and appreciation and relief gave me so much energy that for those first 48 hours I really felt as if I was done with death and pain, and even loss, and that I had for some unknown reason been very very lucky. I was filled with a surety that everything was going to be all right, in just those indeterminate phrases. But it was downhill from there.

On the morning of the third day, the pain returned home bringing all of its kinfolk. Not that any single one of them was overwhelming, but just that all in concert, or even in small repertory groups, they were excruciating. There were constant ones and intermittent ones. There were short sharp and long dull and various combinations of the same ones. The muscles in my back and right shoulder began to screech as if they'd been pulled apart and now were coming back to life slowly and against their will. My chest wall was beginning to ache and burn and stab by turns. My breast which was no longer there would hurt as if it were being squeezed in a vise. That was perhaps the worst pain of all, because it would come with a full complement of horror that I was to be forever reminded of my loss by suffering in a part of me which was no longer there. I suddenly seemed to get weaker rather than stronger. The euphoria and numbing effects of the anesthesia were beginning to subside.

My brain felt like grey mush—I hadn't had to think much for the past two days. Just about the time that I started to feel the true quality of the uphill climb before me—of adjustment to a new body, a new time span, a possible early death—the pains hit. The pain grew steadily worse and I grew more and more furious because nobody had ever talked about the physical pain. I had thought the emotional and psychological pain would be the worst, but it was the physical pain that seemed to be doing me in, or so I wrote at that time.

Feeling was returning to the traumatized area at the same time as I was gradually coming out of physical and emotional shock. My voices, those assorted pieces of myself that guided me between the operations were settling back into their melded quieter places, and a more and more conscious part of me was struggling for ascendancy, and not at all liking what she was finding/feeling.

In a way, therefore, the physical pain was power, for it kept that conscious part of me away from the full flavour of my fear and loss, consuming me, or rather wearing me down for the next two weeks. That two week period of time seems like an age to me now, because so many different changes passed through me. Actually the course of my psychic and physical convalescence moved quite quickly.

I do not know why. I do know that there was a tremendous amount of love and support flowing into me from the women around me, and it felt like being bathed in a continuous tide of positive energies, even when sometimes I wanted a bit of negative silence to complement the pain inside of me.

But support will always have a special and vividly erotic set of image/meanings for me now, one of which is floating upon a sea within a ring of women like warm bubbles keeping me afloat upon the surface of that sea. I can feel the texture of inviting water just beneath their eyes, and do not fear it. It is the sweet smell of their breath and laughter and voices calling my name that gives me volition, helps me remember I want to turn away from looking down. These images flow quickly, the tangible floods of energy rolling off these women toward me that I converted into power to heal myself.

There is so much false spirituality around us these days, calling itself goddess-worship or "the way." It is false because too cheaply bought and little understood, but most of all because it does not lend, but rather saps, that energy we need to do our work. So when an example of the real power of healing love comes along such as this one, it is difficult to use the same words to talk about it because so many of our best and most erotic words have been so cheapened.

Perhaps I can say this all more simply; I say the love of women healed me.

It was not only women closest to me, although they were the backbone. There was Frances. Then there were those women whom I love passionately, and my other friends, and my acquaintances, and then even women whom I did not know.

In addition to the woman energy outside of me, I know that there must have been an answering energy within myself that allowed me to connect to the power flowing. One never really forgets the primary lessons of survival, if one continues to survive. If it hadn't been for a lot of women in my lifetime I'd have been long dead. And some of them were women I did-n't even like! (A nun; the principal of my high school; a boss.)

I had felt so utterly stripped at other times within my life for very different reasons, and survived, so much more alone than I was now. I knew if I lived I could live well. I knew that if the life spark kept burning there would be fuel; if I could want to live I would always find a way, and a way that was best for me. The longer I survive the more examples of that I have, but it is essentially the same truth I knew the summer after my friend Genevieve died. We were sixteen.

To describe the complexities of interaction between the love within and the love without is a lifetime vocation.

Growing up Fat Black Female and almost blind in america requires so much surviving that you have to learn from it or die. Gennie, rest in peace. I carry tattooed upon my heart a list of names of women who did not survive, and there is always a space left for one more, my own. That is to remind me that even survival is only part of the task. The other part is teaching. I had been in training for a long time.

After I came home on the fifth day after surgery, the rest of those two weeks were permeated with physical pain and dreams. I spent the days mostly reading and wandering from room to room, or staring at blank walls, or lying outdoors in the sun staring at the insides of my eyelids. And finally, when at last I could again, masturbating.

Later, as the physical pain receded, it left room for the other. But in my experience, it's not true that first you cry. First you hurt, and then you cry.

For me, there was an important interim period between the actual event and my beginning to come to terms emotionally with what having cancer, and having lost a breast, meant and would mean to my life. The psychic self created a little merciful space for physical cellular healing and the devastating effects of anesthesia on the brain. Throughout that period, I kept feeling that I couldn't think straight, that there was something wrong with my brain I couldn't remember. Part of this was shock, but part of it was anesthesia, as well as conversations I had probably absorbed in the operating room while I was drugged and vulnerable and only able to record, not react. But a friend of mine recently told me that for six months after her mother died, she felt she couldn't think or remember, and I was struck by the similarity of the sensations.

My body and mind had to be allowed to take their own course. In the hospital, I did not need to take the sleeping pills that were always offered. My main worry from day three onward for about ten more was about the developing physical pain. This is a very important fact, because it is within this period of quasi-numbness and almost childlike susceptibility to ideas (I could cry at any time at almost anything outside of myself) that many patterns and networks are started for women after breast surgery that encourage us to deny the realities of our bodies which have just been driven home to us so graphically, and these old and stereotyped patterns of response pressure us to reject the adventure and exploration of our own experiences, difficult and painful as those experiences may be.

On the second day in the hospital I had been crying when the head nurse came around, and she sent in another woman from down the hall who had had a mastectomy a week ago and was about to go home. The woman from down the hall was a smallbodied feisty redhead in a pink robe with a flower in her hair. (I have a permanent and inexplicable weakness for women with flowers in their hair.) She was about my own age, and had grown kids who, she said, wanted her to come home. I knew immediately they must be sons. She patted my hand and gestured at our bandages.

"Don't feel bad," she said, "they weren't that much good anyway." But then she threw open her robe and stuck out her almost bony chest dressed in a gay printed pajama top, saying, "Now which twin has the Toni?" And I had to laugh in spite of myself, because of her energy, and because she had come all the way down the hall just to help make me feel better.

The next day, when I was still not thinking too much, except about why was I hurting more and when could I reasonably expect to go home, a kindly woman from Reach for Recovery came in to see me, with a very upbeat message and a little prepared packet containing a soft sleep-bra and a wad of lambswool pressed into a pale pink breast-shaped pad. She was 56 years old, she told me proudly. She was also a woman of admirable energies who clearly would uphold and defend to the death those structures of a society that had allowed her a little niche to shine in. Her message was, you are just as good as you were before because you can look exactly the same. Lambswool now, then a good prosthesis as soon as possible, and nobody'll ever know the difference. But what she said was, "*You'll* never know the difference," and she lost me right there, because I knew sure as hell *I'd* know the difference.

"Look at me," she said, opening her trim powder-blue man-tailored jacket and standing before me in a tight blue sweater, a gold embossed locket of no mean dimension provocatively nestling between her two considerable breasts. "Now can you tell which is which?"

I admitted that I could not. In her tight foundation garment and stiff, up-lifting bra, both breasts looked equally unreal to me. But then I've always been a connoisseur of women's breasts, and never overly fond of stiff uplifts. I looked away, thinking, "I wonder if there are any black lesbian feminists in Reach for Recovery?"

I ached to talk to women about the experience I had just been through, and about what might be to come, and how were they doing it and how had they done it. But I needed to talk with women who shared at least some of my major concerns and beliefs and visions, who shared at least some of my language. And this lady, admirable though she might be, did not.

"And it doesn't really interfere with your love life, either, dear. Are you married?"

"Not anymore," I said. I didn't have the moxie or the desire or the courage maybe to say, "I love women."

"Well, don't you worry. In the 6 years since my operation I married my second husband and buried him, god bless him, and now I have a wonderful friend. There's nothing I did before that I don't still do now. I just make sure I carry an extra form just in case, and I'm just like anybody else. The silicone ones are best, and I can give you the names of the better salons."

I was thinking, "What is it like to be making love to a woman and have only one breast brushing against her?"

I thought, "How will we fit so perfectly together ever again?"

I thought, "I wonder if our love-making had anything to do with it?"

I thought, "What will it be like making love to me? Will she still find my body delicious?"

And for the first time deeply and fleetingly a groundswell of sadness rolled up over me that filled my mouth and eyes almost to drowning. My right breast represented such an area of feeling and pleasure for me, how could I bear never to feel that again?

The lady from Reach for Recovery gave me a book of exercises which were very very helpful to me, and she showed me how to do them. When she held my arm up to assist me, her grip was firm and friendly and her hair smelled a little like sun. I thought what a shame such a gutsy woman wasn't a dyke, but they had gotten to her too early, and her grey hair was dyed blond and heavily teased.

After she left, assuring me that Reach for Recovery was always ready to help, I examined the packet she had left behind.

The bra was the kind I was wearing, a soft front-hooking sleep-bra. By this time, the Ace bandage was off, and I had a simple surgical bandage taped over the incision and the one remaining drain. My left breast was still a little sore from having been biopsied, which is why I was wearing a bra. The lambswool form was the strangest part of the collection. I examined it, in its blush-pink nylon envelope with a slighter, darker apex and shaped like a giant slipper-shell. I shuddered at its grotesque dryness. (What size are you, she'd said. 38D I said. Well I'll leave you a 40C she said.)

I came around my bed and stood in front of the mirror in my room, and stuffed the thing into the wrinkled folds of the right side of my bra where my right breast should have been. It perched on my chest askew, awkwardly inert and lifeless, and having nothing to do with any me I could possibly conceive of. Besides, it was the wrong color, and looked grotesquely pale through the cloth of my bra. Somewhere, up to that moment, I had thought, well perhaps they know something that I don't and maybe they're right, if I put it on maybe I'll feel entirely different. I didn't. I pulled the thing out of my bra, and my thin pajama top settled back against the flattened surface on the right side of the front of me.

I looked at the large gentle curve my left breast made under the pajama top, a curve that seemed even larger now that it stood by itself. I looked strange and uneven and peculiar to myself, but somehow, ever so much more myself, and therefore so much more acceptable, than I looked with that thing stuck inside my clothes. For not even the most skillful prosthesis in the world could undo that reality, or feel the way my breast had felt, and either I would love my body one-breasted now, or remain forever alien to myself.

Then I climbed back into bed and cried myself to sleep, even though it was 2:30 in the afternoon.

On the fourth day, the other drain was removed. I found out that my lymph nodes had shown no sign of the spread of cancer, and my doctor said that I could go home on the following day, since I was healing so rapidly.

I looked down at the surgical area as he changed the dressing, expecting it to look like the ravaged and pitted battlefield of some major catastrophic war. But all I saw was my same soft brown skin, a little tender-looking and puffy from the middle of my chest up into my armpit, where a thin line ran, the edges of which were held closed by black sutures and two metal clamps. The skin looked smooth and tender and untroubled, and there was no feeling on the surface of the area at all. It was otherwise quite unremarkable, except for the absence of that beloved swelling I had come so to love over 44 years, and in its place was the strange flat plain down across which I could now for the first time in my memory view the unaccustomed bulge of my rib-cage, much broader than I had imagined it to be when it had been hidden beneath my large breasts. Looking down now on the right side of me I could see the curve of the side of my stomach across this new and changed landscape.

I thought, "I wonder how long it was before the Dahomean girl Amazons could take their changed landscapes for granted?"

I cried a few times that day, mostly, I thought, about inconsequential things. Once I cried though simply because I hurt deep down inside my chest and couldn't sleep, once because it felt like someone was stepping on my breast that wasn't there with hobnailed boots.

I wanted to write in my journal but couldn't bring myself to. There are so many shades to what passed through me in those days. And I would shrink from committing myself to paper because the light would change before the word was out, the ink was dry.

In playing back the tapes of those last days in the hospital, I found only the voice of a very weakened woman saying with the greatest difficulty and almost unrecognizable:

> September 25th, the fourth day. Things come in and out of focus so quickly it's as if a flash goes by; the days are so beautiful now so golden brown and blue; I wanted to be out in it, I wanted to be glad I was alive, I wanted to be glad about all the things I've got to be glad about. But now it hurts. Now it hurts. Things chase themselves around inside my eyes and there are tears I cannot shed and words like cancer, pain, and dying.

Later, I don't want this to be a record of grieving only.
I don't want this to be a record only of tears. I want it to
be something I can use now or later, something that I can
remember, something that I can pass on, something that I
can know came out of the kind of strength I have that
nothing nothing else can shake for very long or equal.

My work is to inhabit the silences with which I have
lived and fill them with myself until they have the sounds
of brightest day and the loudest thunder. And then there
will be no room left inside of me for what has been except
as memory of sweetness enhancing what can and is to be.

I was very anxious to go home. But I found also, and
couldn't admit at the time, that the very bland whiteness of
the hospital which I railed against and hated so, was also a kind
of protection, a welcome insulation within which I could
continue to non-feel. It was an erotically blank environment
within whose undifferentiated and undemanding and infan-
talizing walls I could continue to be emotionally vacant—psychic mush—without being required by myself or anyone to be
anything else.

Going home to the very people and places that I loved
most, at the same time as it was welcome and so desirable, also
felt intolerable, like there was an unbearable demand about to
be made upon me that I would have to meet. And it was to be
made by people whom I loved, and to whom I would have to
respond. Now I was going to have to begin feeling, dealing,
not only with the results of the amputation, the physical
effects of the surgery, but also with examining and making my
own, the demands and changes inside of me and my life. They
would alter, if not my timetable of work, at least the relative
pieces available within that timetable for whatever I was
involved in or wished to accomplish.

For instance, there were different questions about time that
I would have to start asking myself. Not, for how long do I

stand at the window and watch the dawn coming up over Brooklyn, but rather, how many more new people do I admit so openly into my life? I needed to examine and pursue the implications of that question. It meant plumbing the depths and possibilities of relating with the people already in my life, deepening and exploring them.

The need to look death in the face and not shrink from it, yet not ever to embrace it too easily, was a developmental and healing task for me that was constantly being sidelined by the more practical and immediate demands of hurting too much, and how do I live with myself one-breasted? What posture do I take, literally, with my physical self?

I particularly felt the need—craved the contact, really—of my family, that family which we had made of friends, which for all its problems and permutations was *my* family, Blanche and Clare and Michelle and Adrienne and Yolanda and Yvonne and Bernice and Deanna and Barbara and Beverly and Millie, and then there were the cousins and surely Demita and Sharon and them, even Linda, and Bonnie and Cessie and Cheryl and Toi with her pretty self and Diane and even my sister Helen. All through that time even the most complicated entanglements between other family members—and there were many not having to do directly with me—all those entanglements and fussings and misunderstandings and stubbornesses felt like basic life-pursuits, and as such were, no matter how annoying and tiresome, fundamentally supportive of a life force within me. The only answer to death is the heat and confusion of living; the only dependable warmth is the warmth of the blood. I can feel my own beating even now.

In that critical period the family women enhanced that answer. They were macro members in the life dance, seeking an answering rhythm within my sinews, my synapses, my very bones. In the ghost of my right breast, these were the micro members from within. There was an answering rhythm in the ghost of those dreams which would have to go in favor of those which I had some chance of effecting. The others had lain around unused and space-claiming for a long time anyway, and at best needed to be re-aired and re-examined.

For instance, I will never be a doctor. I will never be a deep-sea diver. I may possibly take a doctorate in etymology, but I will never bear any more children. I will never learn ballet, nor become a great actress, although I might learn to ride a bike and travel to the moon. But I will never be a millionaire nor increase my life insurance. I am who the world and I have never seen before.

Castaneda talks of living with death as your guide, that sharp awareness engendered by the full possibility of any given chance and moment. For me, that means being—not ready for death—but able to get ready instantly, and always to balance the "I wants" with the "I haves." I am learning to speak my pieces, to inject into the living world my convictions of what is necessary and what I think is important without concern (of the enervating kind) for whether or not it is understood, tolerated, correct or heard before. Although of course being incorrect is always the hardest, but even that is becoming less important. The world will not stop if I make a mistake.

And for all that, I wish sometimes that I had still the myth of having 100 years in this frame, and this hunger for my sister stilled.

Women who speak with my tongue are lovers; the woman who does not parry yet matches my thrust, who will hear; the woman I hold in my arms, the woman who arms me whole...

I have found that people who need but do not want are far more difficult to front than people who want without needing, because the latter will take but sometimes give back, whereas the former simply absorb constantly while always looking away or pushing against and taking at the same time. And that is a wasting of substance

through lack of acknowledgement of both our energies,
and waste is the worst. I know this because I have done
them both.

Coming home from the hospital, it was hard not to feel like a pariah. There were people who avoided me out of their own pain or fear, and others who seemed to expect me to suddenly become someone other than who I have always been, myself, rather than saint or Buddha. Pain does not mellow you, nor does it ennoble, in my experience. It was hard not to feel pariah, or sometimes too vulnerable to exist. There were women who were like the aide in the hospital who had flirted so nicely with me until she heard my biopsy was positive. Then it was as if I had gone into purdah; she only came near me under the strictest of regulatory distance.

The status of untouchable is a very unreal and lonely one, although it does keep everyone at arm's length, and protects as it insulates. But you can die of that specialness, of the cold, the isolation. It does not serve living. I began quickly to yearn for the warmth of the fray, to be good as the old even while the slightest touch meanwhile threatened to be unbearable.

The emphasis upon wearing a prosthesis is a way of avoiding having women come to terms with their own pain and loss, and thereby, with their own strength. I was already dressed to go home when the head nurse came into my room to say goodbye. "Why doesn't she have a form on?" she asked Frances, who by this time was acknowledged by all to be my partner.

"She doesn't want to wear it," Frances explained.

"Oh you're just not persistent enough," the head nurse replied and then turned to me with a let's-have-no-nonsense-now look, and I was simply too tired. It wasn't worth the effort to resist her. I knew I didn't look any better.

At home I wept and wept and wept, finally. And made love to myself, endlessly and repetitively, until it was no longer tentative.

Where were the dykes who had had mastectomies? I wanted to talk to a lesbian, to sit down and start from a common language, no matter how diverse. I wanted to share dyke-insight, so to speak. The call went out. Sonny and Karyn came to the house that evening and the four of us shared our fears and our stories across age and color and place and difference and I will be forever grateful to Sonny and Karyn.

"Take it easy," Sonny said. "Remember you're not really as strong now as you feel." I knew what she meant because I could tell how easily I fell apart whenever I started to believe my own propaganda and overdo anything.

But still she told me about her going to an educational conference three weeks after her surgery, and that she thought now that it probably had been a mistake. But I knew why she had done it and so did she, and we both speechlessly acknowledged that she would probably do it again. It was the urge, the need, to work again, to feel a surge of connection begin with that piece of yourself. To be of use, even symbolically, is a necessity for any new perspective of self, and I thought of that three weeks later, when I knew I needed to go to Houston to give a reading, even though I felt weak and inadequate.

I will also be always grateful to Little Sister. My brother-in-law, Henry, who lives in Seattle and whom I had not seen for seven years, was working in Virginia and had come up to New York to see my mother, passing through Philadelphia where he had grown up to pick up his youngest sister who was called Little Sister, actually Li'l Sister.

Li'l Sister had been quite a hell-raiser in her younger days, but now was an established and matronly black lady of Philadelphia with a college-bound son and rimless glasses. I had never met her before but she knew my mother quite well. When they got to New York my mother told Henry and Li'l Sister that I had had a mastectomy and was home just now from the hospital, so they decided to drop by and see me on their way back to Philadelphia which is only 1 ½ hours south of Staten Island.

Over the phone my mother said to me, with the slightest air of reproach in her voice, "I didn't know all these years that Li'l Sister had had that same operation!" Li'l Sister had had a mastectomy 10 years ago, and neither her brother nor her in-laws had known any thing about it.

Henry is one of the gentlest men I have ever met, although not the most tactful. "Howya doing, girl?" he said, giving me a kiss and settling down to his beer.

I welcomed Li'l Sister, we shared perfunctory remarks and inquiries about each other's children, and very soon the three of us were seated around the dining room table, Henry with his hat and his beer, Li'l Sister proper, reticent and elegantly erect, and me, rather disheveled in a lounging robe. Li'l Sister and I were deeply and busily engaged in discussing our surgeries, including pre- and post-mastectomy experiences. We compared notes on nurses, exercises, and whether or not cocoa-butter retarded black women's tendencies to keloid, the process by which excess scar tissue is formed to ward off infection.

At one point brother Henry sort of wrinkled up his nose and said plaintively, "Can't y'all talk about somethin' else now? Ya kinda upsettin' my stomach."

Li'l Sister and I just looked at him for a moment, and then returned to our conversation. We disagreed about prostheses, but she was very reassuring, and told me what to look out for, like rainy days and colds in the chest. We did every thing but show each other our scars.

At the end of an hour, having refused another cup of tea, Li'l Sister got up, smoothed down her jacket and adjusted her glasses.

"Well, it's been real nice to meet you, Audre," she said, "I've sure enjoyed talking with you. C'mon, Henry, we have to get back to Philly, now."

And they left. Somehow, I had the distinct feeling that she

had never talked to anyone about her mastectomy before, for 10 years. I could be wrong.

Even propped up on pillows I found I couldn't sleep more than three or four hours at a time because my back and shoulder were paining me so. There were fixed pains, and moveable pains, deep pains and surface pains, strong pains and weak pains. There were stabs and throbs and burns, gripes and tickles and itches. I would peep under the bandage when I changed it; the scar still looked placid and inoffensive, like the trussed rump of a stuffed goose, and once the stitches were out, even the puffiness passed.

I would sleep for a few hours and then I would get up, go to the john, write down my dreams on little scraps of paper without my glasses, take two aspirin, do my hand exercises, spider-crawling up the wall of the bathroom, and then go back to bed for another few hours and some more dreams.

I pretty much functioned automatically, except to cry. Every once in a while I would think, "what do I eat? how do I act to announce or preserve my new status as temporary upon this earth?" and then I'd remember that we have always been temporary, and that I had just never really underlined it before, or acted out of it so completely before. And then I would feel a little foolish and needlessly melodramatic, but only a little.

On the day after the stitches came out and I got so furious with the nurse who told me I was bad for the morale of the office because I did not wear a prosthesis, I wrote in my journal:

October 5, 1978
I feel like I'm counting my days in milliseconds, never mind hours. And it's a good thing, that particular consciousness of the way in which each hour passes, even if it is a boring hour. I want it to become permanent. There is so much I have not said in the past few days, that can

only be lived now—the act of writing seems impossible to me sometimes, the space of time for the words to form or be written is long enough for the situation to totally alter, leaving you liar or at search once again for the truth. What seems impossible is made real/tangible by the physical form of my brown arm moving across the page; not that my arm cannot do it, but that something holds it away.

In some way I must aerate this grief, bring heat and light around the pain to lend it some proportion, and god knows the news is nothing to write home about—the new pope is dead, the yankees won the game...

Later

If I said this all didn't matter I would be lying. I see this as a serious break in my work/living, but also as a serious chance to learn something that I can share for use. And I mourn the women who limit their loss to the physical loss alone, who do not move into the whole terrible meaning of mortality as both weapon and power. After all, what could we possibly be afraid of after having admitted to ourselves that we had dealt face to face with death and not embraced it? For once we accept the actual existence of our dying, who can ever have power over us again?

Now I am anxious for more living to sample and partake of the sweetness of each moment and each wonder who walks with me through my days. And now I feel again the large sweetness of the women who stayed open to me when I needed that openness like rain, who made themselves available.

I am writing this now in a new year, recalling, trying to piece together that chunk of my recent past, so that I, or anyone else in need or desire, can dip into it at will if necessary to find the ingredients with which to build a wider construct. That is an important function of the telling of experience. I am also writing to sort out for myself who I was and was becoming throughout that time, setting down my artifacts, not only for later scrutiny, but also to be free of them. I do not wish to be free from their effect, which I will carry and use internalized in one way or another, but free from having to carry them around in a reserve part of my brain.

But I am writing across a gap so filled with death—real death, the fact of it—that it is hard to believe that I am still so very much alive and writing this. That fact of all these other deaths heightens and sharpens my living, makes the demand upon it more particular, and each decision even more crucial.

Breast cancer, with its mortal awareness and the amputation which it entails, can still be a gateway, however cruelly won, into the tapping and expansion of my own power and knowing.

We must learn to count the living with that same particular attention with which we number the dead.

February 20, 1979

I am often afraid to this day, but even more so angry at having to be afraid, of having to spend so much of my energies, interrupting my work, simply upon fear and worry. Does my incomplete gall bladder series mean I have cancer of the gall bladder? Is my complexion growing yellow again like it did last year, a sure sign, I believe, of the malignant process that had begun within my system? I resent the time and weakening effect of these concerns—they feel as if they are available now for diversion in much the same way the FBI lies are available for diversion, the purpose being to sway us from our appointed and self-chosen paths of action.

I must be responsible for finding a way to handle those concerns so that they don't enervate me completely, or bleed off the strength I need to move and act and feel and write and love and lie out in the sun and listen to the new spring birdsong.

I think I find it in work, being its own answer. Not to turn away from the fear, but to use it as fuel to help me along the way I wish to go. If I can remember to make the jump from impotence to action, then working uses the fear as it drains it off, and I find myself furiously empowered.

Isn't there any other way, I said.

In another time, she said.

28 February 1979

III

Breast Cancer: Power Vs. Prosthesis

On Labor Day, 1978, during my regular monthly self-examination I discovered a lump in my right breast which later proved to be malignant. During my following hospitalization, my mastectomy and its aftermath, I passed through many stages of pain, despair, fury, sadness and growth. I moved through these stages, sometimes feeling as if I had no choice, other times recognizing that I could choose oblivion—or a passivity that is very close to oblivion—but did not want to. As I slowly began to feel more equal to processing and examining the different parts of this experience, I also began to feel that in the process of losing a breast I had become a more whole person.

After a mastectomy, for many women including myself, there is a feeling of wanting to go back, of not wanting to persevere through this experience to whatever enlightenment might the at the core of it. And it is this feeling, this nostalgia, which is encouraged by most of the post-surgical counseling for women with breast cancer. This regressive tie to the past is emphasized by the concentration upon breast cancer as a cosmetic problem, one which can be solved by a prosthetic pretense. The American Cancer Society's Reach For Recovery

Program, while doing a valuable service in contacting women immediately after surgery and letting them know they are not alone, nonetheless encourages this false and dangerous nostalgia in the mistaken belief that women are too weak to deal directly and courageously with the realities of our lives.

The woman from Reach For Recovery who came to see me in the hospital, while quite admirable and even impressive in her own right, certainly did not speak to my experience nor my concerns. As a 44 year old Black Lesbian Feminist, I knew there were very few role models around for me in this situation, but my primary concerns two days after mastectomy were hardly about what man I could capture in the future, whether or not my old boyfriend would still find me attractive enough, and even less about whether my two children would be embarrassed by me around their friends.

My concerns were about my chances for survival, the effects of a possibly shortened life upon my work and my priorities. Could this cancer have been prevented, and what could I do in the future to prevent its recurrence? Would I be able to maintain the control over my life that I had always taken for granted? A lifetime of loving women had taught me that when women love each other, physical change does not alter that love. It did not occur to me that anyone who really loved me would love me any less because I had one breast instead of two, although it did occur to me to wonder if they would be able to love and deal with the new me. So my concerns were quite different from those spoken to by the Reach For Recovery volunteer, but not one bit less crucial nor less poignant.

Yet every attempt I made to examine or question the possibility of a real integration of this experience into the totality of my life and my loving and my work, was ignored by this woman, or uneasily glossed over by her as not looking on "the bright side of things." I felt outraged and insulted, and weak as I was, this left me feeling even more isolated than before.

In the critical and vulnerable period following surgery,

self-examination and self-evaluation are positive steps. To imply to a woman that yes, she can be the 'same' as before surgery, with the skillful application of a little puff of lambswool and/or silicone gel, is to place an emphasis upon prosthesis which encourages her not to deal with herself as physically and emotionally real, even though altered and traumatized. This emphasis upon the cosmetic after surgery reinforces this society's stereotype of women, that we are only what we look or appear, so this is the only aspect of our existence we need to address. Any woman who has had a breast removed because of cancer knows she does not feel the same. But we are allowed no psychic time or space to examine what our true feelings are, to make them our own. With quick cosmetic reassurance, we are told that our feelings are not important, our appearance is all, the sum total of self.

I did not have to look down at the bandages on my chest to know that I did not feel the same as before surgery. But I still felt like myself, like Audre, and that encompassed so much more than simply the way my chest appeared.

The emphasis upon physical pretense at this crucial point in a woman's reclaiming of her self and her body-image has two negative effects:

1. It encourages women to dwell in the past rather than a future. This prevents a woman from assessing herself in the present, and from coming to terms with the changed planes of her own body. Since these then remain alien to her, buried under prosthetic devices, she must mourn the loss of her breast in secret, as if it were the result of some crime of which she were guilty.

2. It encourages a woman to focus her energies upon the mastectomy as a cosmetic occurrence, to the exclusion of other factors in a constellation that could include her own death. It removes her from what that constellation means in terms of her living, and from developing priorities of usage for

whatever time she has before her. It encourages her to ignore the necessity for nutritional vigilance and psychic armament that can help prevent recurrence.

I am talking here about the need for every woman to live a considered life. The necessity for that consideration grows and deepens as one faces directly one's own mortality and death. Self scrutiny and an evaluation of our lives, while painful, can be rewarding and strengthening journeys toward a deeper self. For as we open ourselves more and more to the genuine conditions of our lives, women become less and less willing to tolerate those conditions unaltered, or to passively accept external and destructive controls over our lives and our identities. Any short-circuiting of this quest for self-definition and power, however well-meaning and under whatever guise, must be seen as damaging, for it keeps the post-mastectomy woman in a position of perpetual and secret insufficiency, infantilized and dependent for her identity upon an external definition by appearance. In this way women are kept from expressing the power of our knowledge and experience, and through that expression, developing strengths that challenge those structures within our lives that support the Cancer Establishment. For instance, why hasn't the American Cancer Society publicized the connections between animal fat and breast cancer for our daughters the way it has publicized the connection between cigarette smoke and lung cancer? These links between animal fat, hormone production and breast cancer are not secret. (See G. Hems, in *British Journal of Cancer*, vol. 37, no. 6, 1978.)

Ten days after having my breast removed, I went to my doctor's office to have the stitches taken out. This was my first journey out since coming home from the hospital, and I was truly looking forward to it. A friend had washed my hair for me and it was black and shining, with my new grey hairs glistening in the sun. Color was starting to come back into my face and around my eyes. I wore the most opalescent of my moonstones, and a single floating bird dangling from my right ear in the name of grand asymmetry. With an African kente-cloth tunic and new leather boots, I knew I looked fine, with that brave new-born security of a beautiful woman having come through a very hard time and being very glad to be alive.

I felt really good, within the limits of that grey mush that still persisted in my brain from the effects of the anesthesia.

When I walked into the doctor's office, I was really rather pleased with myself, all things considered, pleased with the way I felt, with my own flair, with my own style. The doctor's nurse, a charmingly bright and steady woman of about my own age who had always given me a feeling of quiet no-nonsense support on my other visits, called me into the examining room. On the way, she asked me how I was feeling.

"Pretty good," I said, half-expecting her to make some comment about how good I looked.

"You're not wearing a prosthesis," she said, a little anxiously, and not at all like a question.

"No," I said, thrown off my guard for a minute. "It really doesn't feel right," referring to the lambswool puff given to me by the Reach For Recovery volunteer in the hospital.

Usually supportive and understanding, the nurse now looked at me urgently and disapprovingly as she told me that even if it didn't look exactly right it was "better than nothing," and that as soon as my stitches were out I could be fitted for a "real form."

"You will feel so much better with it on," she said. "And besides, we really like you to wear something, at least when you come in. Otherwise it's bad for the morale of the office."

I could hardly believe my ears! I was too outraged to speak then, but this was to be only the first such assault on my right to define and to claim my own body.

Here we were, in the offices of one of the top breast cancer surgeons in New York City. Every woman there either had a breast removed, might have to have a breast removed, or was afraid of having to have a breast removed. And every woman there could have used a reminder that having one breast did not mean her life was over, nor that she was less a woman, nor that she was condemned to the use of a placebo in order to feel good about herself and the way she looked.

Yet a woman who has one breast and refuses to hide that fact behind a pathetic puff of lambswool which has no relationship nor likeness to her own breasts, a woman who is attempting to come to terms with her changed landscape and changed timetable of life and with her own body and pain and beauty and strength, that woman is seen as a threat to the "morale" of a breast surgeon's office!

Yet when Moishe Dayan, the Prime Minister of Israel, stands up in front of parliament or on TV with an eyepatch over his empty eyesocket, nobody tells him to go get a glass eye, or that he is bad for the morale of the office. The world sees him as a warrior with an honorable wound, and a loss of a piece of himself which he has marked, and mourned, and moved beyond. And if you have trouble dealing with Moishe Dayan's empty eye socket, everyone recognizes that it is your problem to solve, not his.

Well, women with breast cancer are warriors, also. I have been to war, and still am. So has every woman who had had one or both breasts amputated because of the cancer that is becoming the primary physical scourge of our time. For me, my scars are an honorable reminder that I may be a casualty in the cosmic war against radiation, animal fat, air pollution, McDonald's hamburgers and Red Dye No. 2, but the fight is still going on, and I am still a part of it. I refuse to have my scars hidden or trivialized behind lambswool or silicone gel. I refuse to be reduced in my own eyes or in the eyes of others from warrior to mere victim, simply because it might render me a fraction more acceptable or less dangerous to the still complacent, those who believe if you cover up a problem it ceases to exist. I refuse to hide my body simply because it might make a woman-phobic world more comfortable.

As I sat in my doctor's office trying to order my perceptions of what had just occurred, I realized that the attitude towards prosthesis after breast cancer is an index of this society's attitudes towards women in general as decoration and externally defined sex object.

Two days later I wrote in my journal:

> *I cannot wear a prosthesis right now because it feels like a lie more than merely a costume, and I have already placed this, my body under threat, seeking new ways of strength and trying to find the courage to tell the truth.*

For me, the primary challenge at the core of mastectomy was the stark look at my own mortality, hinged upon the fear of a life-threatening cancer. This event called upon me to re-examine the quality and texture of my entire life, its priorities and commitments, as well as the possible alterations that might be required in the light of that re-examination. I had already faced my own death, whether or not I acknowledged it, and I needed now to develop that strength which survival had given me.

Prosthesis offers the empty comfort of "Nobody will know the difference." But it is that very difference which I wish to affirm, because I have lived it, and survived it, and wish to share that strength with other women. If we are to translate the silence surrounding breast cancer into language and action against this scourge, then the first step is that women with mastectomies must become visible to each other.★ For silence and invisibility go hand in hand with powerlessness. By accepting the mask of prosthesis, one-breasted women proclaim ourselves as insufficients dependent upon pretense. We

---

★particular thanks to Maureen Brady for the conversation which developed this insight.

reinforce our own isolation and invisibility from each other, as well as the false complacency of a society which would rather not face the results of its own insanities. In addition, we withhold that visibility and support from one another which is such an aid to perspective and self-acceptance. Surrounded by other women day by day, all of whom appear to have two breasts, it is very difficult sometimes to remember that I AM NOT ALONE. Yet once I face death as a life process, what is there possibly left for me to fear? Who can every really have power over me again?

As women, we cannot afford to look the other way, nor to consider the incidence of breast cancer as a private nor secret personal problem. It is no secret that breast cancer is on the increase among women in America. According to the American Cancer Society's own statistics on breast cancer survival, of the women stricken, only 50% are still alive after three years. This figure drops to 30% if you are poor, or Black or in any other way part of the underside of this society. We cannot ignore these facts, nor their implications, or their effect upon our lives, individually and collectively. Early detection and early treatment is crucial in the management of breast cancer if those sorry statistics of survival are to improve. But for the incidence of early detection and early treatment to increase, american women must become free enough from social stereotypes concerning their appearance to realize that losing a breast is infinitely preferable to losing one's life. (Or one's eyes, or one's hands....)

Although breast self-examination does not reduce the incidence of breast cancer, it does markedly reduce the rate of mortality, since most early tumors are found by women themselves. I discovered my own tumor upon a monthly breast exam, and so report most of the other women I know with a good prognosis for survival. With our alert awareness making such a difference in the survival rate for breast cancer, women need to face the possibility and the actuality of breast cancer as a reality rather than as myth, or retribution, or terror in the night, or a bad dream that will disappear if ignored. After surgery, there is a need for women to be aware of the possibility of bilateral recurrence, with vigilance rather than terror. This is not a spread of cancer, but a new occurrence in the other breast. Each woman must be aware that an honest acquaintanceship with and evaluation of her own body is the best tool of detection.

Yet there still appears to be a conspiracy on the part of Cancer Inc. to insist to every woman who has lost a breast that she is no different from before, if with a little skillful pretense and a few ounces of silicone gel she can pretend to herself and the watching world—the only orientation toward the world that women are supposed to have—that nothing has happened to challenge her. With this orientation a woman after surgery is allowed no time or space within which to weep, rage, internalize, and transcend her own loss. She is left no space to come to terms with her altered life, not to transform it into another level of dynamic existence.

The greatest incidence of breast cancer in american women appears within the ages of 40 to 55. These are the very years when women are portrayed in the popular media as fading and desexualized figures. Contrary to the media picture, I find myself as a woman of insight ascending into my highest powers, my greatest psychic strengths, and my fullest satisfactions. I am freer of the constraints and fears and indecisions of my younger years, and survival throughout these years has taught me how to value my own beauty, and how to look closely into the beauty of others. It has also taught me to value the lessons of survival, as well as my own perceptions. I feel more deeply, value those feelings more, and can put those feelings together with what I know in order to fashion a vision of and pathway toward true change. Within this time of assertion and growth, even the advent of a life-threatening cancer and the trauma of a mastectomy can be integrated into the life-force as knowledge and eventual strength, fuel for a more dynamic and focussed existence. Since the supposed threat of self-actualized women is one that our society seeks constantly to protect itself against, it is not coincidental that the sharing of this knowledge among women is diverted, in this case by the invisibility imposed by an insistence upon prosthesis as a norm for post-mastectomy women.

There is nothing wrong, per se, with the use of prostheses if they can be chosen freely, for whatever reason, after a woman has had a chance to accept her new body. But usually prostheses serve a real function, to approximate the performance of a missing physical part. In other amputations and with other prosthetic devices, function is the main point of their existence. Artificial limbs perform specific tasks, allowing us to manipulate or to walk. Dentures allow us to chew our food. Only false breasts are designed for appearance only, as if the only real function of women's breasts were to appear in a certain shape and size and symmetry to onlookers, or to yield to external pressure. For no woman wearing a prosthesis can even for one moment believe it is her own breast, any more than a woman wearing falsies can.

Yet breast prostheses are offered to women after surgery in much the same way that candy is offered to babies after an injection, never mind that the end effect may be destructive. Their comfort is illusory; a transitional period can be provided by any loose-fitting blouse. After surgery, I most certainly did not feel better with a lambswool puff stuck in the front of my bra. The real truth is that certain other people feel better with that lump stuck into my bra, because they do not have to deal with me nor themselves in terms of mortality nor in terms of difference.

Attitudes toward the necessity for prostheses after breast surgery are merely a reflection of those attitudes within our society towards women in general as objectified and deperson-alized sexual conveniences. Women have been programmed to view our bodies only in terms of how they look and feel to others, rather than how they feel to ourselves, and how we wish to use them. We are surrounded by media images portraying women as essentially decorative machines of consumer function, constantly doing battle with rampant decay. (Take your vitamins every day and he *might* keep you, if you don't forget to whiten your teeth, cover up your smells, color your grey hair and iron out your wrinkles....) As women, we fight this depersonalization every day, this pressure toward the conversion of one's own self-image into a media expectation of what might satisfy male demand. The insistence upon breast prostheses as 'decent' rather than functional is an additional example of that wipe-out of self in which women are constantly encouraged to take part. I am personally affronted by the message that I am only acceptable if I look 'right' or 'normal,' where those norms have nothing to do with my own perceptions of who I am. Where 'normal' means the 'right' color, shape, size, or number of breasts, a woman's perception of her own body and the strengths that come from that perception are discouraged, trivialized, and ignored. When I mourn my right breast, it is not the appearance of it I mourn, but the feeling and the fact. But where the superficial is supreme, the idea that a woman can be beautiful and one-breasted is considered depraved, or at best, bizarre, a threat to 'morale.'

In order to keep me available to myself, and able to concentrate my energies upon the challenges of those worlds through which I move, I must consider what my body means to me. I must also separate those external demands about how I look and feel to others, from what I really want for my own body, and how I feel to my selves. As women we have been taught to respond with a guilty twitch at any mention of the particulars of our own oppression, as if we are ultimately guilty of whatever has been done to us. The rape victim is accused of enticing the rapist. The battered wife is accused of having angered her husband. A mastectomy is not a guilty act that must be hidden in order for me to regain acceptance or protect the sensibilities of others. Pretense has never brought about lasting change or progress.

Every woman has a right to define her own desires, make her own choices. But prostheses are often chosen, not from desire, but in default. Some women complain it is too much effort to fight the concerted pressure exerted by the fashion industry. Being one-breasted does not mean being unfashionable; it means giving some time and energy to choosing or constructing the proper clothes. In some cases, it means making or remaking clothing or jewelry. The fact that the fashion needs of one-breasted women are not currently being met doesn't mean that the concerted pressure of our demands cannot change that.*

There was a time in America not long ago when pregnant women were supposed to hide their physical realities. The pregnant woman who ventured forth into public had to design and construct her own clothing to be comfortable and attractive. With the increased demands of pregnant women who are no longer content to pretend non-existence, maternity fashion is now an established, flourishing and particular sector of the clothing field.

The design and marketing of items of wear for one-breasted women is only a question of time, and we who are now designing and wearing our own asymmetrical patterns and New Landscape jewelry are certainly in the vanguard of a new fashion!

Some women believe that a breast prosthesis is necessary to preserve correct posture and physical balance. But the weight of each breast is never the same to begin with, nor is the human body ever exactly the same on both sides. With a minimum of exercises to develop the habit of straight posture, the body can accommodate to one-breastedness quite easily, even when the breasts were quite heavy.

---

*particular thanks to Frances Clayton for the conversations that developed this insight.

Women in public and private employment have reported the loss of jobs and promotions upon their return to work after a mastectomy, without regard to whether or not they wore prostheses. The social and economic discrimination practiced against women who have breast cancer is not diminished by pretending that mastectomies do not exist. Where a woman's job is at risk because of her health history, employment discrimination cannot be fought with a sack of silicone gel, nor with the constant fear and anxiety to which such subterfuge gives rise. Suggesting prosthesis as a solution to employment discrimination is like saying that the way to fight race prejudice is for Black people to pretend to be white. Employment discrimination against post-mastectomy women can only be fought in the open, with head-on attacks by strong and self-accepting women who refuse to be relegated to an inferior position, or to cower in a corner because they have one breast.

When post-mastectomy women are dissuaded from any realistic evaluation of themselves, they spend large amounts of time, energy, and money in following any will-o-wisp that seems to promise a more skillful pretense of normality. Without the acceptance of difference as part of our lives, and in a guilty search for illusion, these women fall easy prey to any shabby confidence scheme that happens along. The terror and silent loneliness of women attempting to replace the ghost of a breast leads to yet another victimization.

The following story does not impugn the many reputable makes of cosmetic breast forms which, although outrageously overpriced, can still serve a real function for the woman who is free enough to choose when and why she wears one or not. We find the other extreme reported upon in *The New York Times*, December 28, 1978:

ARTIFICIAL BREAST CONCERN
CHARGED WITH CHEATING

A Manhattan concern is under inquiry for allegedly having victimized cancer patients who had ordered artificial breasts after mastectomies.... The number of women allegedly cheated could not be determined. The complaints received were believed to be "only a small percentage of the victims" because others seemed *too embarrassed to complain.* (italics mine)

Although the company in question, Apres Body Replacement, founded by Mrs. Elke Mack, was not a leader in the field of reputable makers of breast forms, it was given ample publicity on the ABC-TV program, "Good Morning, America" in 1977, and it is here that many women first heard of Apres. What was so special about the promises of this product that it enticed such attention, and so much money out of the pockets of women from New York to Maine? To continue from *The New York Times* article:

Apres offered an "individually designed product that is a total duplicate of the remaining breast," and "worn on the body by use of a synthetic adhesive" supposedly formulated by a doctor.

It is reported that in some cases, women paid up to $600, sight unseen, for this article which was supposedly made from a form cast from their own bodies. When the women arrived to pick up the prosthesis, they received something having no relation or kinship to their own breasts, and which failed to adhere to their bodies, and which was totally useless. Other women received nothing at all for their money.

This is neither the worst nor the most expensive victimization, however. Within the framework of superficiality and pretense, the next logical step of a depersonalizing and woman-devaluating culture is the advent of the atrocity euphemistically called "breast reconstruction." This operation is now being pushed by the plastic surgery industry as the newest "advance" in breast surgery. Actually it is not new at all, being a technique previously used to augment or enlarge breasts. It should be noted that research being done on this potentially life-threatening practice represents time and research money spent—not on how to prevent the cancers that cost us our breasts and our lives—but rather upon how to pretend that our breasts are not gone, nor we as women at risk with our lives.

The operation consists of inserting silicone gel implants under the skin of the chest, usually shortly after a mastectomy and in a separate operation. At an approximate cost of $1500 to $3000 an implant (in 1978), this represents a lucrative piece of commerce for the cancer and plastic surgery industries in this country. There are now plastic surgeons recommending the removal of the other breast at the same time as the mastectomy is done, even where there is no clinically apparent reason.

> It is important when considering subcutaneous mastectomy to plan to do both breasts at the same time.... it is extremely difficult to attain the desired degree of symmetry under these circumstances with a unilateral prosthesis.
>
> R.K. Snyderman, M.D.
> in "What The Plastic Surgeon Has To
> Offer in the Management of Breast Tumors"

In the same article appearing in *Early Breast Cancer, Detection and Treatment*, edited by Stephen Gallegher, M.D., the author states:

The companies are working with us. They will make prostheses to practically any design we desire. Remember that what we are doing in the reconstruction of the female breast is by no means a cosmetic triumph. What we are aiming for is to *allow women to look decent in clothes.* (italics mine).... The aim is for the patient to *look normal and natural when she has clothes on her body.*

Is it any coincidence that the plastic surgeons most interested in pushing breast reconstruction and most involved in the superficial aspects of women's breasts speak the language of sexist pigs? What is the positive correlation?

The American Cancer Society, while not openly endorsing this practice, is doing nothing to present a more balanced viewpoint concerning the dangers of reconstruction. In covering a panel on Breast Reconstruction held by the American Society of Plastic and Reconstructive Surgeons, the Spring, 1978 issue of the ACS *Cancer News* commented:

Breast reconstruction will not recreate a perfect replica of the lost breast, but it will enable many women who have had mastectomies *to wear a normal bra or bikini.* (italics mine)

So, even for the editor of the ACS *Cancer News*, when a woman has faced the dread of breast cancer and triumphed, for whatever space of time, her primary concern should still be whether or not she can wear a *normal bra or bikini.* With unbelievable cynicism, one plastic surgeon reports that for patients with a lessened likelihood of cure—a poor prognosis for survival—*he waits two years before implanting silicone gel into her body.* Another surgeon adds,

> Even when the patient has a poor prognosis, she
> wants a *better quality of life.* (italics mine)

In his eyes, obviously, this better quality of life will come, not through the woman learning to come to terms with her living and dying and her own personal power, but rather through her wearing a 'normal' bra.

Most of those breast cancer surgeons who oppose this practice being pushed by the American Society of Plastic and Reconstructive Surgeons either are silent, or tacitly encourage its use by their attitude toward the woman whom they serve.

On a CBS-TV Evening News Special Report on breast reconstruction in October, 1978, one lone doctor spoke out against the use of silicone gel implantations as a potentially carcinogenic move. But even he spoke of women as if their appearance and their lives were equally significant. "It's a real shame," he said, "when a woman has to choose between her life or her femininity." In other words, with a sack of silicone implanted under her skin, a woman may well be more likely to die from another cancer, but without that implant, according to this doctor, she is not 'feminine.'

While plastic surgeons in the service of 'normal bras and bikinis' insist that there is no evidence of increase in cancer recurrence because of breast reconstructions, Dr. Peter Pressman, a prominent breast cancer surgeon at Beth Israel Medical Center in New York City, has raised some excellent points. Although silicone gel implants have been used in enough nonmalignant breast augmentations to say that the material probably is not, in and of itself, carcinogenic, Dr. Pressman raises a number of questions which still remain concerning these implants after breast cancer.

1. There have been no large scale studies with matched control groups conducted among women who have had post-mastectomy reconstruction. Therefore, we cannot possibly have sufficient statistics available to demonstrate whether

reconstruction has had any negative effect upon the recurrence of breast cancer.

2. It is possible that the additional surgery necessary for insertion of the prosthesis could stir up cancer cells which might otherwise remain dormant.

3. In the case of a recurrence of breast cancer, the recurrent tumor can be masked by the physical presence of the implanted prosthesis under the skin. When the nipple and skin tissue is preserved to be used later in 'reconstruction,' minute cancer cells can hide within this tissue undetected.

Any information about the prevention or treatment of breast cancer which might possibly threaten the vested interests of the american medical establishment is difficult to acquire in this country. Only through continuing scrutiny of various non-mainstream sources of information, such as alternative and women's presses, can a picture of new possibilities for prevention and treatment of breast cancer emerge.

Much of this secrecy is engineered by the American Cancer Society, which has become "the loudest voice of the Cancer Establishment."[1] The ACS is the largest philanthropic institution in the United States and the world's largest non-religious charity. Peter Chowka points out that the National Information Bureau, a charity watchdog organization, listed the ACS among the groups which do not meet its standards. During the past decade, the ACS collected over $1 billion from the american public.[2] In 1977 it had a $176 million fund balance, yet less than 15% of its budget was spent on assisting cancer patients.[3]

Any holistic approach to the problem of cancer is viewed by ACS with suspicion and alarm. It has consistently focussed upon treatment rather than prevention of cancer, and then only upon those treatments sanctioned by the most conserva-

---

[1] Chowka, Peter. "Checking Up On the ACS." *New Age Magazine*, April '80, p. 22.
[2] *Ibid.*
[3] Epstein, Samuel. *The Politics of Cancer.* Anchor Books, New York. 1979. p. 456.

tive branches of western medicine. We live in a profit economy and there is no profit in the prevention of cancer; there is only profit in the treatment of cancer. In 1976, 70% of the ACS research budget went to individuals and institutions with whom ACS board members were affiliated.[4] And of the 194 members of its governing board, one is a labor representative and one is Black. Women are not even mentioned.

The ACS was originally established to champion new research into the causes and the cure of cancer. But by its black-listing of new therapies without testing them, the ACS spends much of its remaining budget suppressing new and unconventional ideas and research.[5] Yet studies from other countries have shown interesting results from treatments largely ignored by ACS. European medicine reports hopeful experiments with immunotherapy, diet, and treatment with hormones and enzymes such as trypsin.[6] Silencing and political repression by establishment medical journals keep much vital information about breast cancer underground and away from the women whose lives it most affects. Yet even in the United States, there are clinics waging alternative wars against cancer and the medical establishment, with varying degrees of success.[7]

Breast cancer is on the increase, and every woman should add to her arsenal of information by inquiring into these areas of 'underground medicine.' Who are its leaders and proponents, and what are their qualifications? Most important, what is their rate of success in the control of breast cancer,[8] and why is this information not common knowledge?

The mortality for breast cancer treated by conventional therapies has not decreased in over 40 years.[9] The ACS and its governmental partner, the National Cancer Institute, have

---

[4] *Ibid.*

[5] Chowka, Peter. p. 23.

[6] Martin, Wayne. "Let's Cut Cancer Deaths In Half." *Let's Live Magazine*, August, 1978. p. 356.

[7] Null, Gary. "Alternative Cancer Therapies." *Cancer News Journal*, vol. 14, no. 4, December, 1979. (International Association of Cancer Victims and Friends, Inc. publication).

[8] *Ibid.* p. 18.

[9] Kushner, Rose. *Breast Cancer*. Harcourt, Brace & Jovanovitch. 1975. p. 161.

been notoriously indifferent, if not hostile, to the idea of general environmental causes of cancer and the need for regulation and prevention.[10] Since the american medical establishment and the ACS are determined to suppress any cancer information not dependent upon western medical bias, whether this information is ultimately useful or not, we must pierce this silence ourselves and aggressively seek answers to these questions about new therapies. We must also heed the unavoidable evidence pointing toward the nutritional and environmental aspects of cancer prevention.

Cancer is not just another degenerative and unavoidable disease of the ageing process. It has distinct and identifiable causes, and these are mainly exposures to chemical or physical agents in the environment.[11] In the medical literature, there is mounting evidence that breast cancer is a chronic and systemic disease. Post-mastectomy women must be vigilantly aware that, contrary to the 'lightning strikes' theory, we are the most likely of all women to develop cancer somewhere else in the body.[12]

Every woman has a militant responsibility to involve herself actively with her own health. We owe ourselves the protection of all the information we can acquire about the treatment of cancer and its causes, as well as about the recent findings concerning immunology, nutrition, environment, and stress. And we owe ourselves this information *before* we may have a reason to use it.

It was very important for me, after my mastectomy, to develop and encourage my own internal sense of power. I needed to rally my energies in such a way as to image myself as a fighter resisting rather than as a passive victim suffering. At all times, it felt crucial to me that I make a conscious commitment to survival. It is physically important for me to be loving

---

[10] Epstein, Samuel. p. 462.

[11] *Ibid.* pp. xv-xvi.

[12] Kushner, Rose. p. 163

my life rather than to be mourning my breast. I believe it is this love of my life and my self, and the careful tending of that love which was done by women who love and support me, which has been largely responsible for my strong and healthy recovery from the effects of my mastectomy. But a clear distinction must be made between this affirmation of self and the superficial farce of "looking on the bright side of things."

Like superficial spirituality, looking on the bright side of things is a euphemism used for obscuring certain realities of life, the open consideration of which might prove threatening or dangerous to the status quo. Last week I read a letter from a doctor in a medical magazine which said that no truly happy person ever gets cancer. Despite my knowing better, and despite my having dealt with this blame-the-victim thinking for years, for a moment this letter hit my guilt button. Had I really been guilty of the crime of not being happy in this best of all possible infernos?

The idea that the cancer patient should be made to feel guilty about having had cancer, as if in some way it were all her fault for not having been in the right psychological frame of mind at all times to prevent cancer, is a monstrous distortion of the idea that we can use our psychic strengths to help heal ourselves. This guilt trip which many cancer patients have been led into (you see, it *is* a shameful thing because you could have prevented it if only you had been more. . .) is an extension of the blame-the-victim syndrome. It does nothing to encourage the mobilization of our psychic defenses against the very real forms of death which surround us. It is easier to demand happiness than to clean up the environment. The acceptance of illusion and appearance as reality is another symptom of this same refusal to examine the realities of our lives. Let us seek 'joy' rather than real food and clean air and a saner future on a liveable earth! As if happiness alone can protect us from the results of profit-madness.

Was I wrong to be working so hard against the oppressions

afflicting women and Black people? Was I in error to be speaking out against our silent passivity and the cynicism of a mechanized and inhuman civilization that is destroying our earth and those who live upon it? Was I really fighting the spread of radiation, racism, woman-slaughter, chemical invasion of our food, pollution of our environment, the abuse and psychic destruction of our young, merely to avoid dealing with my first and greatest responsibility—to be happy? In this disastrous time, when little girls are still being stitched shut between their legs, when victims of cancer are urged to court more cancer in order to be attractive to men, when 12 year old Black boys are shot down in the street at random by uniformed men who are cleared of any wrong-doing, when ancient and honorable citizens scavenge for food in garbage pails, and the growing answer to all this is media hype or surgical lobotomy; when daily gruesome murders of women from coast to coast no longer warrant mention in *The N.Y. Times*, when grants to teach retarded children are cut in favor of more billion dollar airplanes, when 900 people commit mass suicide rather than face life in america, and we are told it is the job of the poor to stem inflation; what depraved monster could possibly be always happy?

The only really happy people I have ever met are those of us who work against these deaths with all the energy of our living, recognizing the deep and fundamental unhappiness with which we are surrounded, at the same time as we fight to keep from being submerged by it. But if the achievement and maintenance of perfect happiness is the only secret of a physically healthy life in america, then it is a wonder that we are not all dying of a malignant society. The happiest person in this country cannot help breathing in smokers' cigarette fumes, auto exhaust, and airborne chemical dust, nor avoid drinking the water, and eating the food. The idea that happiness can insulate us against the results of our environmental madness is a rumor circulated by our enemies to destroy us.

And what Woman of Color in america over the age of 15 does not live with the knowledge that our daily lives are stitched with violence and with hatred, and to naively ignore that reality can mean destruction? We are equally destroyed by false happiness and false breasts, and the passive acceptance of false values which corrupt our lives and distort our experience.

The idea of having a breast removed was much more traumatic for me before my mastectomy than after the fact, but it certainly took time and the loving support of other women before I could once again look at and love my altered body with the warmth I had done before. But I did. In the second week after surgery, on one of those tortuous night rounds of fitful sleep, dreams, and exercises, when I was moving in and out of physical pain and psychic awareness of fear for my life and mourning for my breast, I wrote in my journal:

> In a perspective of urgency, I want to say now that I'd give anything to have done it differently—it being the birth of a unique and survival-worthy, or survival-effective perspective. Or I'd give anything not to have cancer and my beautiful breast gone, fled with my love of it. But then immediately after I guess I have to qualify that—there really are some things I wouldn't give. I wouldn't give my life, first of all, or else I wouldn't have chosen to have the operation in the first place, and I did. I wouldn't give Frances, or the children, or even any one of the women I love. I wouldn't give up my poetry, and I guess when I come right down to it I wouldn't give my eyes, nor my arms. So I guess I do have to be careful that my urgencies reflect my priorities.
>
> Sometimes I feel like I'm the spoils in a battle between good and evil, right now, or that I'm both sides doing the fighting, and I'm not even sure of the outcome nor the terms. But sometimes it comes into my head, like right now, what would you really give? And it feels like, even just musing, I could make a

terrible and tragic error of judgement if I don't always keep my head and my priorities clear. It's as if the devil is really trying to buy my soul, and pretending that it doesn't matter if I say yes because everybody knows he's not for real anyway. But I don't know that. And I don't think this is all a dream at all, and no, I would not give up love.

Maybe this is the chance to live and speak those things I really do believe, that power comes from moving into whatever I fear most that cannot be avoided. But will I ever be strong enough again to open my mouth and not have a cry of raw pain leap out?

I think I was fighting the devil of despair within myself for my own soul.

When I started to write this article, I went back to the books I had read in the hospital as I made my decision to have a mastectomy. I came across pictures of women with one breast and mastectomy scars, and I remembered shrinking from these pictures before my surgery. Now they seemed not at all strange or frightening to me. At times, I miss my right breast, the actuality of it, its presence, with a great and poignant sense of loss. But in the same way, and just as infrequently, as I sometimes miss being 32, at the same time knowing that I have gained from the very loss I mourn.

Right after surgery I had a sense that I would never be able to bear missing that great well of sexual pleasure that I connected with my right breast. That sense has completely passed away, as I have come to realize that that well of feeling was within me. I alone own my feelings. I can never lose that feeling because I own it, because it comes out of myself. I can attach it anywhere I want to, because my feelings are a part of me, my sorrow and my joy.

I would never have chosen this path, but I am very glad to be who I am, here.

30 March 1979

Remembering Audre Lorde

The photographs of Audre Lorde on the following pages were all taken by Jean Weisinger at the "I Am Your Sister" Conference in Boston, 1990.

Except where otherwise noted, the written tributes to Audre Lorde were originally published in Sojourner: The Women's Forum, *February 1993, Vol 18. no. 6. We thank the authors for their kind permission in allowing their tributes to be reprinted here.*

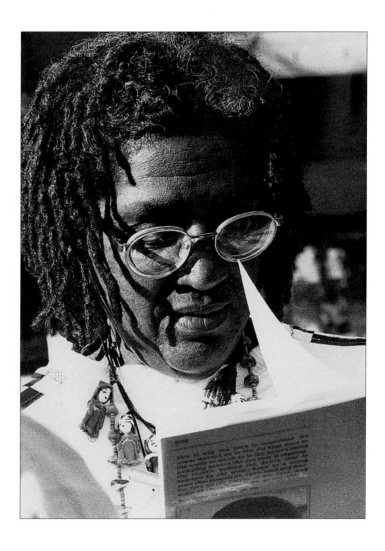

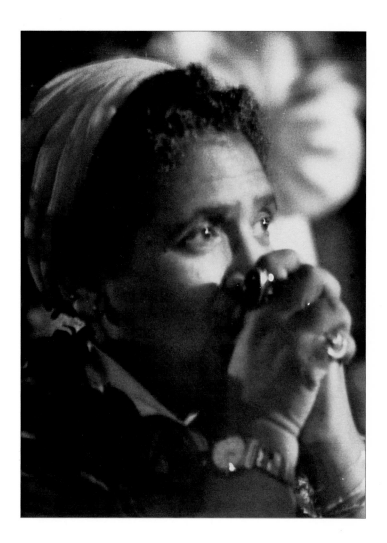

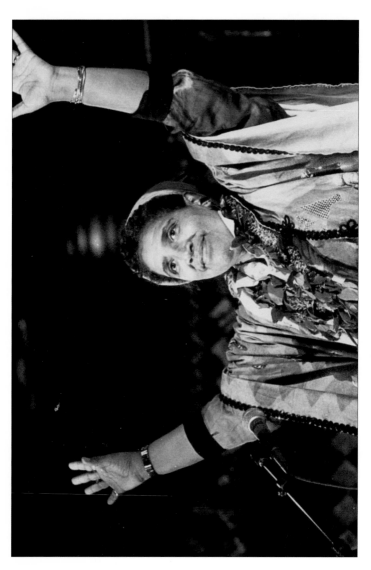

Opening speech, I Am Your Sister, Boston, 1990

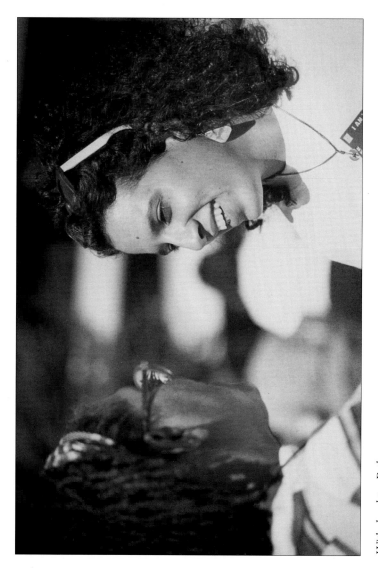

With daughter, Beth

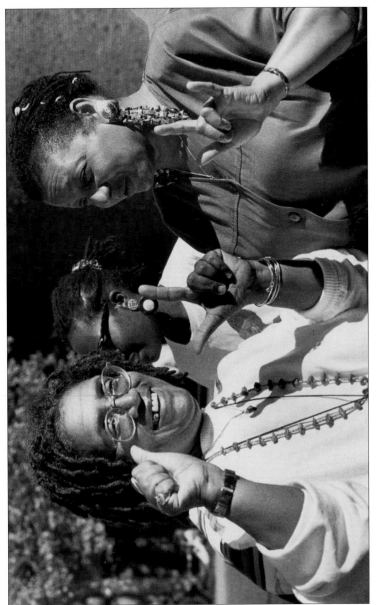

With Shirley Childress Johnson

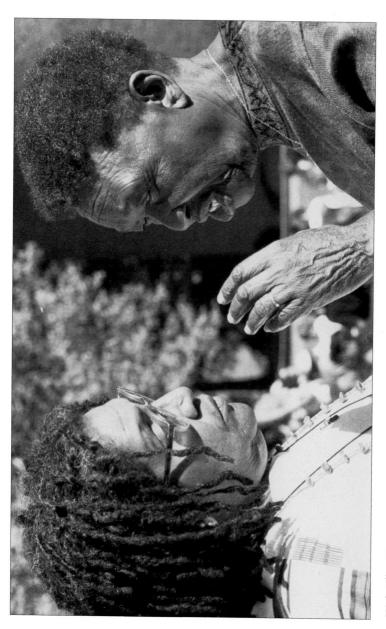

With Ellen Kuzwayo

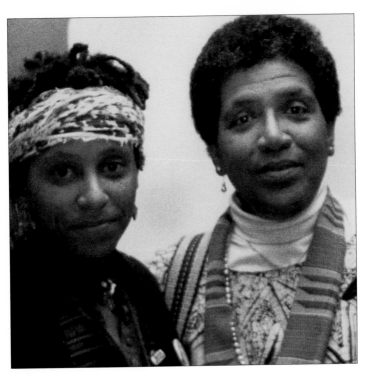

Audre Lorde with photographer, Jean Weisinger, 1988

Remembering Audre

When Audre spoke
She summoned Earth and Sky
Fierce
Her tongue a ringing bell,
Yes
Thunderclap of words.

Audre
Workin' out love and pain
Head up high, face to the sun,
Ceremonious, imperious, raucous
Audre
Dancing her lungs loose
On the heartbeat of womanlove
Audre
Shapeshifting pain into the wit
Of survival
Balm of compassion
Audre
Inventing biomythography.

She was a black lesbian mother warrior
High priestess
Drumming fiery earthcore in poems.
She was a hard rain rolling across the consciousness of America
relentless
She was a strong, loving hand reaching back
To pull us over the hardest parts of ourselves.

Drumbeat Meteorflash Audre Lorde!

Sisters, Brothers,
A prayer, America:
May Audre's example be our biggest dare.

Margaret E. Cronin, *teacher/writer/lesbian/feminist activist,
Arlington, MA.*

What I am taking from Audre Lorde's death is an absolute commitment to fearlessness. I am working toward eradicating fear completely from my life. I think this is necessary because so much of Black women's existence is shackled to fear. Fear of speaking, fear of laughing, fear of crying, fear of shattering silences, fear of being rejected, fear of being seen and, perhaps worst of all, fear of being loved.

If I am to be loved (the right way), then I need to let go of fear and allow those who might come toward me (and my work) really to see me and the complexity of my life as a Black lesbian. I know that I am much more fragile and delicate than I appear to be. I would like to emulate Audre's courage and conviction, by coming into full possession of myself. That means letting everything show—both the big parts of me and the small.

Audre gave oppressed people everywhere a mirror and a voice through which we could see and speak the truth about our lives. She was a gift to the universe. Because of her life and her death, I intend to learn how to be a gift to myself. And hopefully to others who are ready to lay the burden of silence down.

Evelyn C. White, *editor of the* Black Women's Health Book, *Oakland, CA.*

Audre Lorde was a great poet because she understood the necessity of poetry to our collective life and because she knew that beauty and bearing witness to the harsh materials of human struggle need never contradict each other. Across the world, poets, readers, activists are in her debt, for the light shed by her blazing images. The power of her essays and speeches derives directly from her poetic language, her knowledge of "the difference between poetry and rhetoric."

My personal debt to Audre begins over twenty years ago when I found *The First Cities* in the City College of New York (CCNY) bookstore and realized that this extraordinary new poet was also a colleague, someone I could actually talk with. For most of those years, we exchanged drafts of poems, criticized and helped to sustain each other's work. For Audre, there was never any boundary between art and politics, and many of my poems were honed in response to her keenly furthering questions. From the other side, it was always an excitement to receive a bundle of Audre's new drafts and see where her vision and craft were evolving. In the last months of her life, she was working on the poems to be published posthumously as *The Marvelous Arithmetics of Distance*, some of them as remarkable as anything she'd written. She was also working on the subtle and inspired revisions of earlier poems that appear in *Undersong*.

Poetry was at the core of Audre's expressive life, her way of knowing. She helped me trust that in myself, not give way or consent to the marginalizing of that precious resource. In her words: "Poetry is the way we give name to the nameless so it can be thought." This resource nourished her as teacher, activist, witness, breaker of silences, leader, survivor, in all the passages of her life, and in her dying, when she asked me to send her books of poetry. "Poetry is not a luxury," she wrote; and she meant it for all of us.

Adrienne Rich's *latest book is* What is Found There: Notebooks on Poetry and Politics *(W.W. Norton). Santa Cruz, CA.*

To speak of Audre Lorde as a "writer" or an "activist" seems narrow and inadequate. Each of us who read her work or worked with her will have a much more specific and immediate image that will resonate more deeply than categories. For me, Audre has always been a signpost or a lighthouse. She used her words to point toward new paths, new ways of choosing to be in the world.

In the poem "Now That I Am Forever with Child" (1963, in *Undersong*), Audre writes about the birth of her daughter. The final lines are: "I can only distinguish/ one thread within running hours/ you flowing through selves/ toward You." In those words she claimed me, too, as her child and insisted at the same time that I make my own way. She embraced me and pushed me out of the nest. And it was a push I needed; one we all need.

In recent years, I have often been afraid to hear news of her health. After fourteen years of fighting cancer, the end always seemed just at the corner. Whenever I'd receive those calls—she was not doing well—a single image always popped into my mind: the first time I ever saw Audre close up, not at a reading. We, along with hundreds of thousands of others, were at the first Lesbian and Gay Pride March on Washington. I was resting within the throngs on damp grass, amidst a sea of white faces, feeling both exhilarated and lonely. I looked up and there she was, several dozen feet away, talking to a group of women. She was unmistakable in her gele, standing above the mostly sitting crowd. I watched, happy simply to recognize her.

Then she looked up with those piercing, impish eyes. I was just one face among the thousands, but she caught my eye and she winked as if she could see how much I needed that connection just then. It was a flirtatious wink, a sisterly wink, a maternal wink all at once. With it, she took me into her heart, her world, and opened a way for me to be on my own.

In the poem "Prologue" (1971, in *Undersong*) she wrote: "I speak without concern for the accusations/ that I am too much or too little woman/ that I am too Black or too white/ or too much myself...." Audre's genius resided in her insistence on bringing her whole self to whatever she was doing. To be Black, Mother, Lesbian, Poet, Warrior was her art. In doing so, she gave me history for my nourishment and the thrill of the many new ways of being I might choose. Her writing will keep winking at me through the crowd of faces.

Jewelle L. Gomez, *author of* The Gilda Stories, *San Francisco, CA. (A form of this piece originally appeared in* New Directions for Women, *Jan–Feb 1993, as well as in* Sojourner.*)*

Somewhere in the landscape past noon,
I shall leave a dark print of the me that I am.
(from "Prologue," *Chosen Poems: Old & New*)

...we must be very strong
and love each other
in order to go on living
(from "Equinox," *Chosen Poems: Old & New*)

Words sit heavy on my heart, grind against my teeth and tongue like grit, irritate the tender flesh of my eyes like tears uncried. I want to speak words of celebration and remembrance, want them to slide like well-oiled pearls of poetry from my mouth, for she deserves no less. Her words touched me, moved me, inspired me to act, and all I can do is sit here, reading through her books, trying to comfort the huge tremors inside, an earthquake of loss.

Audre Lorde recently adapted the African name Gamba Adisa, which means "warrior, she who makes her meaning known," and that name conveys so much of who this woman was, how her words and ideas strongly defended the reality of all on this planet, how she sought to build bridges between communities with the brick and cable of her words. Her essays and speeches compiled in the volume *Sister Outsider*, as far as I am concerned, form the preeminent textbook of lesbian feminist theory. "Poetry Is Not a Luxury" exhorts women to

> *constantly encourage ourselves and each other to attempt*
> *the heretical actions that our dreams imply, and so many*
> *of our old ideas disparaged.... If what we need to dream,*
> *to move our spirits most deeply and directly toward and*
> *through promise, is discounted as a luxury, then we give*
> *up the core—the fountain—of our power, our woman-*
> *ness; we give up the future of our worlds.*

In "The Transformation of Silence into Language and Action," she observes,

> *I have come to believe over and over again that what is*
> *most important to me must be spoken, made verbal and*
> *shared, even at the risk of having it bruised or misunder-*
> *stood. That the speaking profits me, beyond any other*
> *effect.... [F]or it is not difference which immobilizes us,*
> *but silence.*

One of the most volcanic essays written by Lorde was "The Uses of the Erotic: The Erotic as Power," which elevated the contemporary discourse on eroticism and pornography to a deeper and richer contemplation of the power that women have been systematically taught to discount.

> *The erotic is a resource within each of us that lies in a*
> *deeply female and spiritual plane, firmly rooted in the*
> *power of our unexpressed or unrecognized feeling....*
> *[T]he erotic is not a question only of what we do, it is a*
> *question of how acutely and fully we can feel in the*
> *doing.... [T]he erotic [is] an assertion of the life force of*
> *women, of that creative energy empowered....*

For me personally, calculating the profound effect of living in a time when I was able to hear Lorde deliver her essays and speeches and recite/sing her poems is something analogous to trying to count the myriad stars in our galaxy on my fingers. Some core reality of my being a writer, a lesbian feminist essayist, poet, novelist, and performance artist is a plant grown from seeds scattered by the fertile tree of life that Lorde nurtured and tended by her very being, for her writing and speaking and surviving were a living example for me of what possibilities we all hold inside. I never dreamed I could be a poet. I never imagined that my words would touch the lives of others. Lorde lived a life that helped me to understand that such goals were attainable in this life. Her grace and courage in facing the cancer in her body gave me the strength to deal with the disabilities that diminish my own physical reality. Her willingness to address the things that divide us from each other and to offer thoughtful suggestions of ways to heal the wounds in our community inspired my own creative consideration of how we can better live together in this world, fully conscious of our privileges and responsibilities.

The Grand Canyon exists as a huge chasm in the earth, worn away by centuries of water eroding tiny grains of sand and stone. The Hope Diamond was created from centuries of pressure by the earth squeezing atoms of carbon into their rarefied form. I was not witness to the process that created either of these magnificent examples of applied power. However, I have been alive and present and witness to such power in action in the life of Audre Lorde. Long after all of us now alive are atoms in the universal void, some magnificent reminder of the greatness she represented will inspire awe in future generations.

Ayofemi Folayan, *lesbian feminist journalist, creative writing teacher, and community activist, Los Angeles, CA.*

꩜

It started to rain. It hasn't rained all month and today after reading that Audre Lorde is dead, it rains. I move from the steps where I am sitting and go stand up under the tree.

Last night I stayed up almost the entire night hoping there would maybe be something about her death on the news. Maybe CNN, I thought, watching the TV almost all night before falling asleep. There was nothing, or maybe they announced her death after I fell asleep.

I remember when James Baldwin died. It was on the news, and they had an article in our paper about him and his life. There was also a last interview from him in *Essence* magazine. Someone wrote a biography. The shelves of our library were once again filled with all the books James Baldwin had ever written. There was even some poetry that he had written.

Will they do the same for Audre Lorde? I think, standing there under the tree getting soaked. I wonder, maybe in New York or Boston or some other big city, there'll be articles written or a documentary or something? Maybe someone will even write a biography. No. Maybe they won't, I think, leaning up against the tree, feeling the rain fall through the branches.

I should have stayed on the steps, because standing here under the tree is no protection. There's never really any protection anyway. Lorde knew that. That's what she always knew. That regardless of what fear of what pain, there is never any protection but the strength that you gain from knowing you have to live. Out, in the light, visible before the world. Or die underneath behind trees getting soaked anyway. That's what her work said to me. Thank you, Audre Lorde. Thank you.

Linda Cue, *Black Feminist Writer, Gainesville, FL.*

I grew up by the Mississippi River. Hell, for most of my life I've lived within 70 miles of that river. Not next to her, mind you—I never lived in a river town. But *by* her. Not close enough to know her intimately: her daily changes, her seasons, her little sounds, or those people closest to her. But close enough to know her power, to feel the constant tug of her mystery, to have the very way I understand my world shaped by her presence just off to the west. Every time I get close to the Mississippi now, more often in memory than not, I long for whatever it is that, from deep within her, pulls deep within me.

There are women who, to me, are also that river—runnin alongside my life, pullin me in. Audre Lorde has been, and is, one of these women, flowin through my life a mile wide and a continent long.

There's a word for loving something we've never touched: hope.

Elliott, *34 year-old Radical Feminist Dyke writer and activist, Philadelphia, PA.*

Audre, everything seems more fragile since you're gone. You gave us so much strength of purpose, not only with your work or in your heroic struggle with cancer but out of the weave of both those offerings, the way you moved them in and with and through one another. The way you pulled at lost strands of history and made them sing. It was what you said and how you made sure you filled each diminishing breath in a way that would be useful to us all: such a rare and powerful legacy.

When you died, my first emotion was almost one of relief. Such an arduous battle, so many days and weeks and months of suffering. If I truly sat with it, the loss seemed overwhelming. But I chose to envision you at peace. Then, too, the poems and essays reassured me; they remain to comfort and to go on teaching. It's only in the last few days that this enormous sense of fragility has set in. Suddenly I know the world is a more dangerous place, our lives more precarious, with you gone.

Tasting this fragility, Minister Malcolm comes to mind. As you were so aware of everything going on around you, I'm sure you know a revival of interest in Malcolm's life surged just before you died. Barbara and I saw Spike Lee's film and left the theater in a kind of daze, unwilling even to voice criticism of one aspect of the rendition or another. We were too busy experiencing the texture and the meaning of an era and a man that had helped shape who we are.

And that's when I began to understand what happens when great teachers are taken from us—by bullets or cancer or whatever the enemy hones to murder the best among us. Like Malcolm, you have done your job—a thousandfold. Now it's up to each of us to figure out how to take what you've given and use it, every day of our lives. If we do not, this sense of fragility will invade our cells, move in to stay.

So, dear Sister, rest for a while—if you can. It's been a hard one. But I imagine you already seeing with your eyes, hearing with your ears, laughing again your great contagious laugh, touching with your exquisite sensitivity, pulling deep knowledge and honest feeling together once more, on the next journey's wings.

Margaret Randall, *author of* Gathering Rage: A Failure of 20th Century Revolutions to Develop a Feminist Agenda. *Albuqurque, NM.*

When I read in the newspaper about the death of Audre Lorde, the Great Plains wind was howling at the windows. I tried to think of someone I could call, just another woman I could connect to here in the Heartland, someone to help ease the loss. I dreaded the likely response: "Who was she?"

There are not many here in the Heartland who recognize her name, but there are more than a few who recognize the words: "The master's tools will never dismantle the master's house." These are words many women in the Heartland/Bible Belt struggle with. We struggle with the reality of those words and with the imperative fed to us on a daily basis that if we stray from the master's words, we will be annihilated.

I stared for a long time at the death notice in the newspaper. As darkness fell, the wind continued howling. I lit a few candles and lay awake for most of the night, staring at the shadows on the walls and listening to the wind. I thought, "This is the Goddess Audre not ready to leave, singing her last song," and I felt safe, comforted somehow, knowing in a new way that her words would live on.

The next afternoon I met for coffee with someone I rarely see—one of the "ladies." She commented that I seemed a little down. When I told her Audre Lorde had died, her face crumbled and she tried unsuccessfully to hold back tears in her eyes. "I know her work," she said, "and I carry it in my heart." And I realized the meaning of her statement here in the Heartland Bible Belt Rape Capital of America, where the message to remain silent is laced with violence. I realized there are many kinds of activism—public and private. Audre Lorde's words have affected many women in personal and private ways, ways that have enabled survival in the face of patriarchal oppression in its most redneck good ol' boy form.

There will be only one Audre Lorde. But when the wind howls, when spring brings new life and a woman anywhere carries Lorde's words in her heart, we will know the Goddess is always with us.

Elizabeth Sargent, *poet and activist, Norman, OK.*

I became acquainted with Audre Lorde on a personal basis through correspondence. When attempting to put together an anthology, I asked her to contribute an essay. In her letter to me of June 7, 1975, she expressed trepidations: "I'm a poet not an essayist." Nevertheless, she did. As a result, I like to think that I had a small part in encouraging her to consider another genre. She went on to write some of the most courageous, insightful and trailblazing prose of this century, bestowing a new dimension to African-American and women's literature. It is sad that one who had so much to give and gave so much, has passed too soon. She will certainly be missed. Her voice, however, will continue to be heard in her words. Audre left to us her spear for women warriors.

Ann Allen Shockley, *novelist, Nashville, TN.*

The first thing is the writing. That was what mattered to her most. Audre was one of the most gifted writers of our generation, not just in this country, but the world. Since childhood she'd worked to hone her craft to a point of absolute precision, to create a uniquely beautiful and always indentifiable voice. She succeeded. The woman could really write.

The despicable irony is that because she also always insisted upon telling the truth with her words, to reveal, as she would say, the texture of what it meant to be a "Black, lesbian, mother, warrior, woman," Audre's writing, for all the honors it received, never got the full recognition it deserved.

We had a lifetime conversation about the ostracism that she and all Black lesbians and gay men face when we have the courage to come out and to name homophobia as the political issue it is. Those conversations were always angry, often sardonic, and sometimes the tears were just beneath the surface.

Here was a woman who was born and raised in Harlem, who incorporated African cultures in her life and art long before the term Afrocentric even existed, and who challenged racism *wherever* she found it, and who was still a "sister outsider" in relationship to the Black cultural and political establishment because she had the integrity to say out loud and in print that she loved women.

The author of ten books of poetry and four books of prose, Audre was never satisfied merely to build a brilliant career, because in tandem with her art she was equally committed to freedom. Audre understood that in order for her work as an African-American woman, a lesbian, a feminist to make any sense at all, she had to do something to alter the actual political context in which that writing would be read. This was the understanding that led her to cofound SISA: Sisterhood in Support of Sisters in South Africa and Kitchen Table: Women of Color Press. This was what motivated her, even when she was in Berlin this summer to get alternative cancer treatment, to write a letter to Helmut Kohl protesting racist violence against "immigrants" who happen to be people of color. She was the kind of artist, of which there are fewer and fewer, who took political responsibility for using her gifts to bring about revolutionary change.

Meeting Audre in 1976 undoubtedly changed my life. As a graduate student who was teaching myself Black literature, who was trying to carve out a space for Black women writers, who named myself a Black feminist when the term was considered an anathema, and who had recently come out as a Black lesbian, which insured pariah status even more certainly than it does today, meeting Audre changed my life.

One of Audre's gifts to me was what she wrote and said about feelings, how essential it is to explore, acknowledge, and use not only emotions but intuition and spiritual insights to create art, a movement, a world fundamentally different from anything that white/male constructs have been able to conceive. She knew that a politic that only addressed issues from the neck up, no matter how theoretically "correct," would never work to liberate women of color, the world's majority.

Undoubtedly, it was her ability to name her feelings, to nurture and reveal her soul that helped her to survive and flourish for so long. She dealt with breast cancer like every other challenge in her life: wrote about it, made herself an expert on it, and used it to expand not just her own, but many other's understandings. She beat back death so many times that we sometimes thought she'd outsmarted it once and for all. Now that she's gone we have her words:

> I trace the curve of your jaw
> with a lover's finger
> knowing the hardest battle
> is only the first
> how to do what we need for our living
> with honor and in love
> we have chosen each other
> and the edge of each other's battles
> the war is the same
> if we lose
> someday women's blood will congeal
> upon a dead planet
> if we win
> there is no telling
> (From "Outlines," *Our Dead Behind Us*)

Barbara Smith, *cofounder of Kitchen Table: Women of Color Press. Albany, NY.*

(An edited version of this obituary appeared in the December 1 issue of The Village Voice *as well as in* Sojourner.*)*

The last time I saw Audre, she said to me, "Last week I was dying, but now I'm not." I was dying, but now I'm not. I have never met anyone who was more self-possessed and self-determined than Audre Lorde. She looked fiercely within herself, she looked fiercely at people and the world around her, and she called it like she saw it. How wonderful that Audre, who was once a little girl who did not talk much and could not see well, born in Harlem during the Depression, determined herself to become one of the most visionary, outspoken, and eloquent writers of our time.

There are many of us who work hard and have many special skills and talents. We write, we speak, we go to countless meetings, we work hard to be educated and to take care of our families, we give our time and labor for things we believe in; we contribute. I think you'd agree that there are few people who do all of these things and who are also able to speak to and move so many different kinds of people as Audre. She brought us together, not only here in the United States but also in Canada, Europe, and Australia. She brought us together in Berlin, Soweto, Amsterdam, and St. Croix. She brought us together, women and men, Black and White and Asian and Latina and Indigenous, all sexualities and class backgrounds. Audre brought us together even when we weren't so sure that's where we wanted to be.

"I am Black, Feminist, Lesbian, mother, warrior, woman, lover, poet doing my work." This straightforward, seemingly simple act of naming herself and her purpose, wherever she found herself, required great will, focus, and courage. Audre was able to claim each part of her identity with such authority because she had paid the price. She paid the price by walking into the fire of self-examination and self-disclosure. She looked at herself and showed herself, however painful those acts.

A few weeks after Audre's death, a small group of mostly Black Lesbians in the Boston area gathered together, as people did all over the country and throughout the world, to remember Audre, to read her work, and to talk about the influence she had on our lives. One quality that was mentioned over and over was Audre's generosity. There was story after story of how Audre would answer letters, send cards and unsolicited checks, write references and recommendations. She served on committees, boards and panels. She traveled to meet with groups of women when she didn't feel well. She apologized when she realized she was wrong.

I first met Audre and read with her in Boston during the summer of 1979 when Barbara Smith and others organized an evening of Black women's poetry with Fahamisha Brown, Diana Christmas, and a number of others to raise money for the Women's Safety Committee in the wake of the murders of twelve Black women. The following evening Audre and Adrienne Rich gave a big reading at Harvard University. A Black woman journalist had come to the reading to interview Audre for an article she was submitting to the now defunct, supposedly progressive, *Real Paper*. Audre, in true Audre fashion, encouraged the interviewer to talk to women from the area, which she did. Needless to say, the editors were not interested in running a story about unpublished, local Black women writers. It didn't matter. What mattered was Audre's expansive, far-seeing vision. She was generous with her time, her talents, her power, her money, her influence, her humor, and her love. She was generous with her energy, her sexiness, and her expertise. But, more than that, Audre was generous with her explorations into her own fears and angers, her own mortality.

Most of my contact with Audre continued to be at events connected to writing: the *Sojourner*/Kitchen Table Benefit, the International Feminist Book Fair in Montreal, the I Am Your Sister Conference in Boston in 1990 to honor her work. One of the experiences I cherish most was attending the 1989

Oberlin College graduation with a group of us from the Boston area. After a poweful introduction by Chandra Mohanty, Audre delivered the commencement address and received an honorary degree. All of this had special significance to me because I had first gone to that campus twenty years before as an undergraduate, at a time when calling a meeting for ourselves as Black women or coming out as Lesbian or Gay, especially for people of color, was dangerous and frightening, a grim event. That day, when Audre spoke, the Lesbian, Gay and Bisexual students, including the Third World Lesbian and Gay organization, staged an action, asking everyone to wear pink armbands. Most of the Black graduating students wore red, black, and green hoods with their gowns. The class president's address was delivered by a Black Gay and the valedictory address was delivered by a Black man who wore a pink armband. Times had changed because of Audre and so many others, and I was glad to be there to see it.

That day, Audre asked us the question that she had asked herself: Are you willing to use the power that you have in the service of what you say you believe? It's a brilliant question, a crucial question, because it includes everyone, lets no one off the hook. She asks us to consider and to choose. The question is empowering because it assumes that each one of us has some kind of power, regardless.

Audre, in her complete generosity of spirit, cleared a space for us to be. She cleared a space for Black Lesbians that has never existed in the world before. Now we are called upon to think more deeply, to speak louder, to work harder, to be more of ourselves, to keep our claim on the space that Audre cleared. We have been blessed to have Audre in our lives. And, best of all, because of her, we have each other.

Precious Audre. We miss her. But there is something we must always remember: We, here, are as precious as Audre. Anything we would hesitate to say to Audre, we best rethink before we say to each other. Anything we regret not saying to her, we best say to each other. Anything we wish we had done for her, we best do for each other.

Precious Audre. She was dying, now she's not.
Precious Audre. You were dying, now you're not.

Kate Rushin *delivered a lengthier version of this rememberance December 11, 1992, at a memorial for Audre Lorde held at English High School in Jamaica Plain, MA. The event was sponsored by the Women's Theological Center. Kate Rushin is the author of* The Black Back-Ups *(Firebrand).*

Praisesong for the Poet
for Audre Lorde
by Kate Rushin

Drummers are always like that
Take it in Put it out Use it
Before she lose it

Drummers are always like that
Flashy Dazzling Cool
Cool not too cool to
Get hot
Get down
Sounds
Her axe
Sounds her creation
Sounds her life
Plangent and sweet sweet
Vibrations pounding resounding
Strikes the sweet spot sweating
Eyeing us over her symbols trembling
Audre Audre

Leaves her body
Her body
This body this body
Lay down bloodbed
Stretch out restbed
Arch up lovebed
Cool sheets for your sickbed
Witness witness
Witness your deathbed this body
This body
Honey brass bell tongue
Kettle of flame
This body this body
Won't come by here again

Leaves her books her words
Her sisters her children her lovers
Her poetry emotion

Audre Audre
Gives us bottom
Keeps Time
Audre Audre
Got to
Give the
Drummer
Some

Audre Lorde (1934–1992)

Audre Lorde was born in New York City on February 18, 1934 to Linda Belmar and Frederick Byron Lorde, immigrants from Grenada. She wrote her first poem when she was in the eighth grade. Lorde started taking courses at Hunter College in New York in 1951, and eventually received her B.A. in 1959. In 1961 she received her Masters of Library Science from Columbia University. After working several years as a librarian, during which time she married and gave birth to her two children, Lorde received an NEA grant in 1968 and became poet-in-residence at Tougaloo College. There she met Frances Louise Clayton, who eventually become her partner of nineteen years. She published her first volume of poetry, *The First Cities*, in 1968. In 1978 she became a professor of English, first at John Jay College of Criminal Justice in New York, and later at Hunter College.

Both her poetry and prose have received numerous honors, including a nomination for the National Book Award for *From a Land Where Other People Live* in 1974, the American Library Association's Gay Caucus Book of the Year Award for *The Cancer Journals* in 1981, the Manhattan Borough President's Award for Excellence in the Arts in 1988, and the American Book Award for *A Burst of Light* in 1989. In October of 1990, Lorde's work and life were celebrated by over a thousand women attending the "I Am Your Sister" conference in Boston.

Audre Lorde died of cancer on November 11, 1992.

Works by Audre Lorde

The First Cities. New York: Poets Press, 1968.

Cables to Rage. London: Breman, 1970.

From a Land Where Other People Live. Detroit: Broadside Press, 1973.

New York Head Shop and Museum. Detroit: Broadside Press, 1974.

Between Our Selves. Point Reyes, CA: Eidolon Editions, 1976.

Coal. New York: Norton, 1976.

The Black Unicorn. New York, Norton, 1978.

Uses of the Erotic: The Erotic as Power. Out & Out Pamphlet. Freedom, CA: Crossing Press, 1978.

The Cancer Journals. San Francisco: Aunt Lute, 1980.

Chosen Poems: Old and New. New York: Norton, 1982.

Zami: A New Spelling of My Name. Freedom, CA: Crossing Press, 1982.

Sister Outsider: Essays and Speeches. Freedom, CA: Crossing Press, 1984.

Apartheid USA and Our Common Cause in the Eighties. Authored jointly with Merle Woo. Freedom Organizing Pamphlet. Latham, NY: Kitchen Table: Women of Color Press, 1986.

I Am Your Sister: Black Women Organizing across Sexualities. Freedom Organizing Pamphlet. Latham, NY: Kitchen Table: Women of Color Press, 1986.

Our Dead Behind Us. New York: Norton, 1986.

A Burst of Light. Ithaca, NY: Firebrand Books, 1988.

Undersong: Chosen.Poems Old and New. New York: Norton, 1992.

The Marvelous Arithmetics of Distance. New York: Norton, 1993.

aunt lute books is a multicultural women's press that has been committed to publishing high quality, culturally diverse literature since 1982. In 1990, the Aunt Lute Foundation was formed as a non-profit corporation to publish and distribute books that reflect the complex truths of women's lives and the possibilities for personal and social change. We seek work that explores the specificities of the very different histories from which we come, and that examines the intersections between the borders we all inhabit.

Please write or phone if you would like us to send you a free catalogue of our other books or if you wish to be on our mailing list for future titles. You may buy books directly from us by phoning in a credit card order or mailing a check with the catalogue order form.

Aunt Lute Books
P.O. Box 410687
San Francisco, CA 94141
(415) 826-1300

This book would not have been possible without the kind contributions of the *Aunt Lute Founding Friends*:

Anonymous Donor	Diana Harris
Anonymous Donor	Phoebe Robins Hunter
Rusty Barcelo	Diane Mosbacher, M.D., Ph.D.
Marian Bremer	William Preston, Jr.
Diane Goldstein	Elise Rymer Turner